WHAT WOMEN ARE SAYING ABOUT NICOLE RONSARD'S PROGRAM

■ *I began Nicole Ronsard's regime in mid-July. By September, without cheating, I knew that her system worked.*

■ *My copy of Nicole Ronsard's book has proved to be about the best investment I have ever made for my looks, my figure, and my energy level.*

■ *I started Nicole's program midsummer. By early winter I noticed with utter amazement that my entire lower body was smoother and firmer than it had been since my teens.*

■ *Thanks to Nicole I have completely changed my lifestyle. After seeing such dramatic improvement in my figure within a few months, no way would I consider going back to my old habits.*

■ *Now I can wear shorts to jog, without embarrassment, thanks to Nicole Ronsard.*

■ *I am a great believer in Nicole Ronsard's philosophy . . . and have had much success in reshaping my body.*

■ *My mother is getting fantastic results from your program. This is a great incentive for me.*

■ *As a salon owner I recommend your book as a prerequisite to my figure-contouring treatments because there's no way I could take away or add to what you have to say.*

■ *Being a health and fitness consultant and exercise teacher, I have made Nicole Ronsard's book required reading for the hundreds of people in my classes.*

Also by Nicole Ronsard

CELLULITE: THOSE LUMPS, BUMPS AND BULGES
YOU COULDN'T LOSE BEFORE

Beyond Cellulite

BEYOND
CELLULITE

Nicole Ronsard's Ultimate

Strategy to Slim, Firm and

Reshape Your Lower Body

NICOLE RONSARD

Villard Books ■ *New York* ■ *1992*

Copyright © 1992 by Nicole Ronsard

All rights reserved under International and Pan-American Copyright Conventions. Published in the United States by Villard Books, a division of Random House, Inc., New York, and simultaneously in Canada by Random House of Canada Limited, Toronto.

Villard Books is a registered trademark of Random House, Inc.

This book contains advice on diet and exercise. Anyone beginning a diet or exercise regime, and anyone commencing the fruit and vegetable cure contained in this book should consult a physician.

Library of Congress Cataloging-in-Publication Data

Ronsard, Nicole.
   Beyond cellulite : Nicole Ronsard's ultimate strategy to slim, firm, and reshape your lower body / Nicole Ronsard.
     p.   cm.
   ISBN 978-0-679-73936-4
   1. Cellulite. 2. Reducing. 3. Nutrition. 4. Exercise.
I. Title.
RM222.R66 1992
646.7'5—dc20   91-58089

Book design by Beth Tondreau Design
Book photography by Jon Van Gorder
Line drawings by Nga Le

146406575

TO MY SON, MY BEST FRIEND

Your courage and your strength have been an inspiration.
You've never brought me anything but joy.

Acknowledgments

- My warmest thanks to my longtime friend Jan Rosenthal, to whom I am forever indebted for her help and support.

- A heartfelt acknowledgment to Rita Ross, who did a wonderful job of organizing and reorganizing a great deal of material.

- A very special thanks to the staff at Villard Books, especially to Diane Reverand for her enthusiasm and vision.

- Last but not least I shall always be grateful to my audience. These many years later, I would like to offer my abiding thanks to the millions of women who read my first book and supported my beliefs through the years.

Preface

t is almost two decades since my first book *Cellulite: Those Lumps, Bumps and Bulges You Couldn't Lose Before* was published. Through these years the issue of cellulite has proven to be much more than a passing fad and has become a well-established concern to American women just as it has been in Europe for years.

Times have changed, women have changed, but cellulite has not. All the diet trends that have come and gone have done little to eradicate this annoying, frustrating and often figure-distorting problem.

Cellulite is definitely more than skin deep. To a large extent it is a clear reflection of our physiology. While my first book was the stepping-stone to a basic understanding of the cellulite condition, in the years since, I have devoted myself to research which, while not altering my initial concepts, has greatly expanded the fundamental theory of cellulite formation and the practical ways to reverse it.

All the material here is brand new and in keeping with the numerous advances in nutrition, fitness and lifestyle that have come into existence in the past decade or so.

True to the promise implied in its title, the new findings presented in *Beyond Cellulite* are formulated for lasting results that reach far beyond the cellulite condition into total fitness and glowing health. A sensible approach to nutrition, exercise, stress management and body care will lead you to the ultimate reward: a firm, smooth, shapely, healthy body that functions at peak efficiency over a lifetime.

Nicole Ronsard
September 1991

Contents

Contributing Factors: Poor Posture ● Sitting and Standing ●
Crossing the Legs ● Wearing High Heels ● Restrictive Garments
■ What About Genetics? ■ The Hormonal Link ■ Cellulite-Forming
Patterns ■ A Final Word About Your Figure . . . and Your Weight

Brushing: How to Do It • Self-Massage: How to Do It • A Few
More Suggestions for Massaging the Body ▪ Air Baths ▪ Avoid
Prolonged Exposure to the Sun ▪ Some Final Tips to Keep Skin Taut
and Youthful

The Mind-Body Connection ▪ Stress: The Invisible Enemy ▪ The
Stress-Cellulite Connection ▪ Some Valuable Tips for Minimizing
Stress ▪ Relaxation Techniques to Help You De-Stress ▪ Visualization:
Visualization Techniques • Additional Visualization Techniques •
Applying Visualization Principles ▪ Affirmations

PART THREE: SOME EXTRA HELP

The Ten-Day Cure: How to Do It ▪ Salt Baths

Introduction: Straight Talk About Cellulite

Cellulite, we all seem to know by now, is every woman's special *bête noire*—well, practically every woman's, if we consider that 90 percent of women over the age of sixteen are affected to some degree by this frustrating figure problem. Since my last book, the condition that we call cellulite has been discussed, analyzed, and even argued about a great deal, and has become a very popular topic among women and in the media. In fact, an entire industry of creams, lotions, and massage mitts has developed to treat cellulite.

It is my intention, here, to give a thorough presentation of all the facts surrounding the cellulite issue. More important, I shall explain in detail how the problem can be eliminated once and for all. One of my strongest beliefs is that every woman can achieve a desirable figure. No matter how advanced your cellulite condition may be, with a commitment to the program I have designed, you can eliminate cellulite or, at the very least, bring it under control.

First, it is necessary to understand all of the circumstances that play a role in the development of cellulite—from the earliest stages to the more advanced or stubborn cases. All of this will be explained in plain language. Once you have discovered what has gone wrong—and I do believe that cellulite represents a "disturbance" of some sort rather than a natural or inevitable tendency—you are then in a position to correct the problem. It is important to keep in mind that cellulite is a *syndrome*, the result of a combination of factors that come into play to produce lumps and bulges in the hip and thigh area. This is why a *systemic*, or *whole body*, approach is required to correct it.

Cellulite has been described repeatedly as nothing more than fat. At this point, I only wish to say that while cellulite is often accompanied by excess weight, such is not always the case. In fact, thin women complain just as much about cellulite, and some who look quite fine in clothing have a very pronounced problem that is all the more frustrating because they have no fat to lose. Cellulite does not seem to discriminate: It can affect women of any size or shape. The beauty of the *Anti-Cellulite Strategy* is that it allows automatically for weight loss in the cases when it is desirable or necessary. For those who have achieved ideal weight, this strategy enables maintenance without effort. When you are *eating right*, you are *feeding* your body rather than starving it into thinness.

Cellulite clearly reflects a *body out of balance*, a body that has somehow lost its natural harmony. Several factors come into play here. In the broadest sense, it is our lifestyle that is responsible. Consider for a moment the abuse our bodies endure on a daily basis. We overeat, we eat on the run without digesting properly, we eat anything that is handy when we are hungry and sometimes even when we are not hungry at all. We surrender to cravings when we know we shouldn't. We drink alcohol and we smoke cigarettes—sometimes for social reasons and other times to cope with stress. The stress that we live with daily takes its toll week by week, year by year. We often lead sedentary lives whether by necessity or by choice. Almost everything we do as adults—sitting at desks, spending our social time in restaurants or at cocktail parties, lounging at the beach or home—can cause problems over a period of time.

In other words, cellulite does not appear overnight. Like wrinkles and like excess fat, it develops gradually, insidiously. Then, one day, we discover to our horror that things are not quite the same as they once were. Rather than give in to panic or depression, what we must do is take charge and set into motion an intelligent course of measures that takes into consideration the physiology of the human body. Working with the body, not against it, is a very important part of this program.

This lack of balance occurs when things are not going quite the way they should, when they are disrupted by errors in lifestyle. Essentially, the disturbance takes place in what the French call the *milieu intérieur*, or internal environment—that is, the true environment of our cells. The internal environment is made up of fluids that bathe all the cells of the body. This fluid medium, which brings nourishment to cells and carries away their waste products, plays a vital role not only in the way we look and feel but also in the way the body ultimately shapes up. What characterizes cellulite is a disturbance of this fluid medium which occupies all the tiny spaces between cells. Two major factors play a role here: *lymphatic circulation*, the slow and steady movement of this fluid, and *tissuemineral balancing*, mainly sodium and potassium. A lack of efficiency in these two functions leads to a form of congestion that is at the root of the cellulite problem.

Our goal is to eliminate this congestion, to get things flowing properly, and thereby smoothe out the characteristic lumps and bumps of the cellulite condition. My Anti-Cellulite Strategy includes proper nutrition, effective exercise, body care, stress management, and visualization. Followed carefully and with dedication, this program is the only *sure* way to reverse a cellulite condition permanently. Unfortunately, to this day there are no miracle cures. As much as we all would like to believe in a pill or a cream or a device, cellulite responds *only* when we treat it from the inside out. But this is not bad news at all. On the contrary, when we make the commitment to eat right, exercise regularly, control stress, and care for our bodies, we do ourselves the biggest possible favor—and we benefit in every way. That is why I have called this book *Beyond Cellulite*. Our ultimate goal is to improve overall health and vitality while smoothing out the lumps, ripples, and bulges. The results will be dramatic and lasting. You will be astounded at achieving such rich rewards for efforts that have become habitual.

I cannot promise that in six weeks or six months your problem will vanish as if by magic. But I *can* promise that if you faithfully follow my suggestions—and I have purposefully made the program very, very flexible—you will be delighted with the results.

Eventually, you will have dissolved all the accumulated cellulite formations, and the new habits that you establish will discourage future formations. You will understand what it means to live beyond cellulite, and the rewards will be manifold. Best of all, you will be in charge of your figure and your health—for the rest of your life.

Part One # CELLULITE UPDATE

1

The Cellulite Syndrome

I n France, where women have been cellulite-conscious for many decades, what we now call cellulite has had, over the years, several other names, including *lipodystrophy* and *hydrolipodystrophy*, which are often used in medical literature, and *graisse parasite* (inactive fat), and *graisse rebelle* (stubborn fat). None of these terms, however, ever quite caught on as did cellulite, which is now part of the universal language of health and beauty, and we shall continue to use it as a descriptive term.

What *cellulite* describes quite simply is the annoying figure problem of lumps and bumps characterized by a dimply, spongy appearance that are generally found in the hip and thigh area. In more pronounced cases, these lumps and bumps take on a puckered look and become the distorting bulges that interfere with normal, graceful body contours.

WHY A "SYNDROME"?

Cellulite is essentially a disturbance in the body's natural chemistry, and this is why it responds to treatment from the *inside out* and not to external methods alone. Even though it forms in the adipose or fatty tissue, cellulite is *not* a special kind of fat. It may or may not be accompanied by excess fat, and even the hinnest and most active women can suffer a cellulite condition. In other words, fat may be part of the cellulite syndrome, but there is a great deal more involved. Many things are happening simultaneously—and that is the nature of a syndrome—to bring about the lack of balance or harmony in the body before we recognize a cellulite problem.

THE KEY FACTORS

There are several factors to consider in the process of cellulite formation. I call these the "key factors." Briefly, they are:

Skin Structure

Right beneath the epidermis or outer layer of skin there is loose, connective tissue made up of: *cells*, predominantly fat cells, which store energy, and fibroblasts, the cells that synthesize collagen; *fibers*, collagen and elastin, a meshlike network that gives the skin support and resiliency; and a *ground substance* or matrix that is gel-like in texture and is the "glue" that holds everything together. Nestled among these components are blood vessels, lymphatics, and nerve endings. A harmonious equilibrium must exist in this layer for the skin to appear smooth and firm. As we shall see, this equilibrium can be easily disrupted.

Location

The cellulite-prone areas, the hips and thighs, are the very areas on a woman's body where the tissue layer is thicker, spongier, and more loosely structured—and thereby allows for more "disruption." Also, if there is excess fat, it tends to accumulate here. This process does not occur randomly but is genetically programmed by our hormones. These are the same hormonal factors that favor water retention, which can further accentuate and aggravate a cellulite problem.

Circulation

When circulation is sluggish in cellulite-prone areas, there results a certain congestion: capillaries weaken and excess seepage takes place, which causes a buildup of fluids in the tiny spaces between cells. The circulation of the capillaries, called *microcirculation*, must function very efficiently for optimal nourishment and minimal fluid stagnation. Improving microcirculation is one of our major goals in the Anti-Cellulite Strategy.

Muscles

A lack of good muscle tone can be a major contributing factor to a cellulite condition. Typically, cellulite develops in those areas where muscles are underused and underdeveloped. For example, a lack of tone in the gluteus, the heavy muscle that supports the buttocks, will cause that muscle to sag, thus accentuating and sometimes creating the characteristic bulge on the upper side of the thigh. By strengthening the gluteal muscles we can "lift" the upper thigh and thereby reduce its sagging and/or bulging appearance.

Nutrition

The quantity of food that we eat is not, by itself, responsible for cellulite. But the *quality* of the food is. A lack of essential nutrients—the result of poor food choices, sloppy eating habits, and other dietary abuses—will, over a period of time, create imbalances at cell level and set off a chain reaction that will lead directly to cellulite. For example, a lack of potassium and/or an excess of sodium is a major contributing factor to the congestion that characterizes cellulite. In the typical diet, sodium intake far outweighs that of potassium, thereby jeopardizing the delicate balance that must be maintained between these two essential minerals. An important part of our nutritional program will be to maximize potassium and minimize sodium to establish a better ratio and correct the deficiency.

Stress

Proper, healthy functioning of the body depends upon efficient physiology—digestion, circulation, breathing, and elimination. Stress can interfere with all of these functions to a greater or lesser degree. In addition, stress adversely affects our endocrine glands, especially the adrenals, which regulate water balance in the body. Stress often leads to overeating and bingeing. In other words, our entire physiology is thrown off balance by stress, tension, and anxiety. Cellulite and premature aging are two of the devastating consequences.

Age

As we get older, and this can start in the early twenties, our connective tissue begins to break down. The skin loses elasticity, especially when we are inactive and/or overweight. While there is not any set age for cellulite to develop, there are patterns that tend to occur at certain times in our lives. For example, in the teen years, poor eating habits can develop. In our twenties and thirties, we may experiment with various trendy diets that contribute to tissue deterioration. Age itself is not an accurate measure for the cellulite pattern; it is the habits that we form at different stages that can lead to cumulative damage.

Gravity

When the tissues have been subjected to repeated variations in volume, mainly through the overuse and abuse of reducing diets, the skin and its underlying support system stretch and give way to the downward pull of gravity. The sagging that results here compounds a cellulite problem and makes it more visible.

TAKING CONTROL IS THE ANSWER

I hope that now you are beginning to understand the *systemic nature* of cellulite and how it develops. I also hope that you are beginning to realize that it is possible to take control of the situation. Because cellulite is chiefly the result of a series of errors in lifestyle, we can alter its course and eventually restore order to a system that has been riddled by abuses. Throughout these chapters, I will explain and demonstrate how you can reverse a cellulite condition as well as prevent it from coming back.

MEN AND CELLULITE

Although cellulite is generally regarded as a women's problem, men can and do develop it. In fact, most adult men struggle with cellulite without giving it a specific name, possibly because, in men, it is not located in the same areas, nor does it have the same appearance, as in women.

The accumulation of fat is programmed by hormones. While excess fat on women accumulates on the hips and thighs, on men it collects above and around the waist. Those fatty deposits, called "love handles," that plague an overwhelming number of men are really a form of cellulite. Surprised? There is no need to be when you consider that men are subject to the same errors in lifestyle that affect their bodies.

Men have connective tissue that is vulnerable to the same physiological changes as women's. Naturally, it makes sense that the same factors, or at least many of the same factors, will lead to the form of congestion that causes cellulite. As we shall see in Chapter 3, poor nutritional habits, sedentariness, stress, poor circulation, and restrictive garments (for some men, a belt worn in the same place for years) will lead to stubborn pockets of fat and cellulite. What's more, these bulges are just as hard for men to lose as women's lumpy hips and thighs.

Even men who exercise regularly and consider themselves to be in good shape will complain vehemently about their love handles. The problem, in short, forms in those areas where muscles are underused and rarely called for in everyday movements. Poor posture certainly does not help and as such can be considered an aggravating factor.

The very fact that these bulges develop on slender men—and are so stubbornly resistant to diet and exercise—confirms that there is more involved here than just plain fat. And when we look into the actual cellulite-forming process and its causes, it seems fairly obvious that this problem can affect men as well as women.

The reason that cellulite has a different appearance on men has to do with the actual structure of their connective tissue. On women, this tissue is looser and there tends to be more of it, while men often escape visible lumpiness because of naturally tighter subcutaneous tissue as well as thicker skin.

So, women are not the exclusive victims of this annoying figure problem. Talk to any man who has struggled in his attempt to get rid of unsightly bulges, and he will express the same exasperation as women who struggle with lumps and bulges on hips and thighs. It seems obvious then that men will benefit equally from an effective program that goes to the root of the problem with dietary measures and other changes in lifestyle.

2

Cellulite Up-Close

LET'S TAKE A PEEK

The human body is quite a remarkable structure. There is no machine, not even the most intricate and highly developed computer, that can function as precisely and purposefully as the human body. And its functions go on twenty-four hours a day, through waking and sleeping, all through our lives. All we are required to do is provide the raw materials and the proper care.

Let's imagine that we can take a peek into the layer of tissue where cellulite forms. If we could do this for even a moment, what we would learn would be not only surprising but extremely beneficial to an understanding of the overall functioning of our physiology.

If we could magnify this tissue layer hundreds of times and then get a good glimpse of it in action, we would see a number of things occurring simultaneously. All of them important in sustaining the life of cells and tissues. For our purpose of understanding the cellulite process, we will look at these functions individually. Of course, this goes on throughout the body, but our focus here is the subcutaneous tissue.

Capillaries

Each of us has about 10 billion capillaries with a total surface area greater than 500 square meters. It is in these tiny vessels that surround cells that the most purposeful function of the circulation occurs, namely the interchange of nutrients and cellular wastes between tissues and circulating blood. When these vital functions are disrupted, the capillaries can weaken and seep more fluid than is desirable into the spaces between cells. This excess seepage is the beginning of the cellulite process.

Tissue Spaces

One-sixth of the body is made up of spaces between cells. Because nutrients pass from blood to cells by a process of diffusion through the liquid medium surrounding each cell, it is essential that cells be close together and that the distances between capillaries and cells be maintained at a minimum. The tiny spaces between cells, the interstitial spaces, should hold no more fluid than is necessary to maintain a healthy, clean "internal environment," one in which the nutrient-waste interchange can take place efficiently. When excess fluid is present, a buildup of viscous material occurs. This, in turn, will spread the cells apart and thereby increase the distances not only between cells but between cells and capillaries. The exchanges then will become more difficult. Congested tissue is inefficient tissue.

The Potassium Factor

It must be appreciated that oxygen and nutrients do not pass directly from capillaries to cells. Rather, they diffuse into the interstitial fluid, and from there they are picked up by the cells. Wastes follow a similar route in reverse. What powers this process to a large extent is the ratio of minerals present in the tissues, namely sodium and potassium. Together, these two minerals form a "pump" that speeds nutrients into the cells while speeding their wastes out. Congestion in the tissues will weaken this very important mechanism, called the "sodium-potassium pump," and slow down the exchanges. Tissue sludge will result, and this will further impair exchanges and lower cell metabolism.

The body should derive a sufficient amount of sodium from a balanced diet of wholesome foods. When we exceed the amount that the body needs—a very common occurrence in the way most people eat today—we have a sodium buildup that, in addition to encouraging water retention, leads to decreased cell activity. Potassium is the mineral that naturally counterbalances sodium. Potassium predominates inside the cells while sodium is found mainly in the fluid surrounding the cells. The better the balance between the two minerals, the more efficient the "pumping" action. When this balance is disrupted by poor eating habits, excess salt in the diet, sedentariness, and stress, among other factors, sodium will draw excess fluids to the tissue spaces. This highly undesirable collection of excess fluids will create congestion, which suppresses or slows down cellular activity, impairs the diffusion of nutrients and oxygen, and hinders cells from repairing and renewing themselves.

Waste Products

Our trillions of cells are ceaselessly at work to nourish, repair, and renew themselves. This ongoing activity, called cell metabolism, generates wastes that must be removed promptly. In every twenty-four-hour period, the average adult loses billions of cells, and these worn-out or dead cells must be eliminated. Undigested or partially digested foods may add to the normal level of wastes. Chemicals we take in from foods, water, the environment, and medications also contribute to the burden of bodily wastes. These wastes lodge themselves everywhere in the body: in our organs, tissues, cells, and in the spaces between cells. When the body is in balance, there is a minimum of these wastes, and they are removed as they form, carried away by the lymph to be filtered and eliminated.

This process, however, does not necessarily occur evenly in the body: In the areas where circulation is particularly sluggish—in this case, the hips, thighs, and buttocks—wastes may accumulate faster than they can be evacuated. When waste products build up, they impede microcirculation to cells and tissues, decreasing the amount of oxygen and nutrients carried to the cells as well as reducing wastes eliminated from the cells. The result is tissue sludge, which further slows cellular activity and eventually manifests itself as lumpy cellulite. We now have a less than ideal situation in our internal environment.

Free Radicals

Free radicals, or oxidation radicals—highly unstable molecules that attack, infiltrate, and injure vital cell structures—are constantly formed in the body as a natural by-product of body chemistry. Environmental pollution contributes to the formation of free radicals and so does "internal pollution." Cigarette smoking, excessive consumption of alcohol and caffeine, drugs, stress, constipation, and illness all increase the body's load of oxidizing substances.

A diet high in fat, along with overeating in general, contributes to the body's burden of free radicals. These molecules are most readily released in fat, and the more food you metabolize, the more free radicals you produce. Burning fat too quickly also causes the release of these damaging molecules, another reason to avoid quick-weight-loss schemes. Commonly, free radicals attack collagen, a major component of connective tissue and the skin's basic support structure, causing it to degenerate and age prematurely. Exposure to the sun is another major source of free radical damage. The damage from free radicals is cumulative and self-perpetuating: free radicals release more free radicals.

Wastes and Body Toxicity

For years, researchers in Europe have pointed out the relationship between cellulite and body toxicity. The incomplete removal of wastes from the colon (constipation) is responsible for a great deal of toxic buildup. Also, women who complain about a cellulite condition often experience sluggishness with their livers and kidneys, two of the major purifying organs. Fatigue is very often an indication of the level of toxicity in our bodies and part of a vicious cycle: fatigue releases toxins, which leads to greater fatigue. Stress and tension also release toxins into our bodies. Finally, we reach an overload of toxicity in our purifying and eliminative organs as well as in the tissue spaces between cells. This overload affects our health, energy, and general vitality along with our figures. Obviously, what is called for here is an overall cleansing of the body at cell level to help the whole system function better.

The All-Important Lymph

The primary function of lymphatic circulation is bodily cleansing. While we all know about arterial and venous circulation, few of us are really familiar with lymphatic circulation. Yet it is vital to health, energy, fitness, and a smooth figure. The circulation of the lymph works in close cooperation with the circulation of the blood, but it is quite different. It functions in part as an adjunct to microcirculation.

Lymph is the fluid that surrounds and bathes all the cells of the body and constitutes the "internal environment" of our cells. Just as we could not survive for very long in a highly polluted, suffocating environment, our cells also require a healthy environment in order to function optimally.

The lymph operates by drawing excess fluids, cellular wastes, and other substances from the spaces between cells and carries them away to "filtering stations" called lymph nodes. These nodes are located at various sites throughout the body. Lymph channels ultimately drain into two large veins near the heart so that lymph is returned to the bloodstream to be further processed and then carried toward the eliminative organs. The lymphatic system has been called the body's "metabolic waste disposal," and it is easy to understand why this expression is appropriate. Of course, this is only one aspect. The lymphatic system serves many other functions, such as guarding against infections and disease. But our focus here is circulation.

Unlike the blood, which is powered by the heart, the lymph has no such central pump or prime mover. Lymphatic circulation relies upon muscular contractions and deep breathing to move it along. It is a naturally slow-moving fluid that circulates, for the most part against gravity, through a vast network of tiny capillaries called lymphatics. These extremely thin-walled vessels run throughout the body but are concentrated in subcutaneous tissue.

The fluid in tissue spaces, the interstitial fluid, is constantly renewed through lymphatic circulation. When it enters the tiny vessels that drain it away, it becomes lymph. For cells to be nourished and for tissues to remain healthy, smooth, and firm, the exchange of nutrients and wastes must occur steadily and without hindrance; cells can carry on efficiently only when their wastes are removed promptly and when no excess water is present.

When the flow of lymph is slowed down, a stagnation of interstitial fluid occurs in the tissues. In areas where circulation tends to be poor and relies almost entirely on gravity to move it back up, as in the hip and thigh area, this stagnation encourages the formation of cellulite. Poor lymphatic circulation also results in fatigue and sluggishness and creates conditions conducive to disease and cell degeneration with its accompanying premature aging. Efficient lymph drainage should be one of our main concerns, not only to help eliminate cellulite but for our health and vitality as well.

Throughout the book, I will show you different ways and techniques to improve lymphatic circulation as well as the quality of the lymph itself.

3

The Various Conditions
That Play a Role

CELLULITE DOES NOT JUST "HAPPEN"

Until now, we have been focusing our attention on the physiological aspects of cellulite. I have presented this simplified "crash course" in physiology because I believe it is extremely important to understand as much as possible about what is happening internally—more precisely, in the layer of tissue where cellulite forms—to bring about the unsightly, externally visible lumps and bumps. If you really desire a smooth, cellulite-free figure, then you will want to arm yourself with as much knowledge as possible.

Now that we have taken a good look at the cellulite condition at close range, we can get down to the business of what we do to cause this problem. Yes, that's right, *we* cause the problem—it does not just *happen* to us. It is important to keep in mind that the human body constantly strives for balance and harmony. We are the ones who upset its delicate mechanisms and rhythms. We sabotage Nature's precision with carelessness.

If I were to make a single statement about cellulite that explains the problem in the broadest terms, I would say that "The way we live is the ultimate cause of cellulite." Once you become aware of all the things we do to create this problem, you will understand the many implications of such a general statement. The main culprits in the cellulite story are *poor eating habits, sedentariness,* and *stress.* Briefly, these three major factors work in the following ways to produce lumps, bumps, and bulges.

Poor Eating Habits

Wrong food choices, day in and day out, add up to serious nutritional deficits. "Convenience," or processed, foods—short on nutrients and rich in fats, sugar, and salt, not to mention the loads of chemicals used in their preparation—form the bulk of most people's diets. Eating in this manner too often precludes fresh fruits and vegetables, which are then relegated to the position of "extras" or side dishes rather than as major parts of the meal. The same is true of beverages: sugary soft drinks and commercial juices prevent us from drinking plenty of pure water.

The *way we eat* also has a great deal to do with figure problems. We frequently eat too fast and without chewing our food properly. This, in turn, leads to indigestion, which has become all too common a problem in our society. The various remedies such as antacids and laxatives only aggravate matters by interfering with efficient physiology. The same is true of such medications as pain killers, tranquilizers, diet pills, and "pep" pills, which we reach for all too easily and too often. These add stress to an already overburdened system. Caffeine, alcohol, and nicotine do the same.

A general lack of discipline in eating leads to another situation, which complicates the cellulite pattern: the overuse and abuse of reducing diets. For many, this has become the norm. Invariably, nutritional deficiencies result. Statistics show that 31 percent of American women between the ages of nineteen and thirty-nine diet at least once a month—and nearly 20 percent consider themselves "perpetual dieters." Other studies indicate that at least half of all adult women and 25 percent of all adult men go on diets two or more times a year.

While people have certainly become more aware of good nutrition in recent years, it is obvious that there is still room for improvement.

Sedentariness

For many of us, sitting for long hours is a daily reality. We often tend to prolong this inactivity in our leisure hours—too much time spent in restaurants, at the movies, watching television, and just sitting around. Many potentially serious problems result: poor circulation, shallow breathing, sluggish lymph flow, and faulty digestion to name a few.

Although many more people are active now, thanks to the fitness movement, studies show that an overwhelming majority of people still get insufficient exercise.

Stress

While most people can easily understand why careless nutrition and lack of exercise could be responsible for cellulite, they find it difficult to realize that tension can be just as responsible. In short, stress, tension, and anxiety play havoc with our bodily systems by interfering with digestion, elimination, circulation, sleep patterns, and energy levels. And it is not just the major upheavals of life that contribute to faulty physiology; slowly but surely daily irritations and annoyances wear us down and do the most damage in the long run.

A MATTER OF LIFESTYLE...

Perhaps you are beginning to see how these errors in lifestyle, repeated over and over, actually set the ground for cellulite to form. These patterns and habits may not take their toll for years, and certainly cellulite does not just appear in the course of a day. The cumulative effect of these abuses will gradually and eventually lead to lumpy cellulite.

SOME OTHER CONTRIBUTING FACTORS

There are a number of other factors that play a role in bringing about the ripples and bulges. Poor circulation, for one, plays a big role in creating the right environment for cellulite to develop and grow. While cellulite seems to collect in areas with poor circulation, once it forms, it compounds the problem even more, thus leading to a sort of vicious cycle. Anything that will slow down or interfere with normal blood flow will act as a contributing factor to cellulite.

Poor Posture

Sitting or walking slouched over compresses the body's organs so that they function less efficiently, and this, in turn, puts additional strain on the circulatory system.

Inactivity

Sitting or standing in one position for extended periods of time causes fluids to "pool" or collect in the lower limbs.

The Various Conditions That Play a Role

Crossing the Legs

Sitting with legs crossed directly interferes with circulation in the lower limbs by putting pressure on the main vein that runs along the inner thigh. This also contributes to the deterioration of this fragile area.

Wearing High Heels

Wearing improper shoes for hours on end constricts the calf muscles and interferes with blood flow. The artificial positioning caused by high heels forces realignment of the entire body.

Restrictive Garments

Wearing tight clothing, belts, and underwear that "cut" into the flesh will cause fluids to collect immediately above or below that point. Over a period of time this will create bulges and dents in the figure. Furthermore, by giving the illusion of support, these garments will bring about a slackening of muscles.

In addition, *pregnancy, premenstrual bloating,* and *constipation* all cause an increase of volume in the lower abdomen and interfere with circulation in the legs.

WHAT ABOUT GENETICS?

While it is true we inherit many things from our parents, it is extremely important to keep in mind that genetically transmitted tendencies and predispositions are quite different from fully developed problems. The fact that one's mother may have cellulite certainly does not doom a woman to the same plight. In fact, awareness of the tendency toward this condition can serve an invaluable asset in counteracting the problem or discouraging its development. While we can do little to change the stature, bone structure, and body frame that are genetically determined, there is a great deal we can do to prevent figure problems such as ripply cellulite.

There is no doubt that we all "inherit" a lifestyle from our families. The attitudes, ideas, and values that we learn at an early age often stay with us through our lives. The way in which food is prepared and eaten is certainly part of this package. So is an attitude toward exercise and other physical activity. In other words, these acquired habits are far more likely to lead us in the direction of developing cellulite than any particular genetic factor or what we call "heredity" and upon which we tend to blame entirely too many things.

THE HORMONAL LINK

Female hormones play a role in creating a setting conducive to cellulite formation by promoting the development of fat and by favoring fluid retention in the hip and thigh area. There are certainly times in a woman's life when hormones are especially active—puberty, pregnancy, menopause—and in some cases, the cellulite-forming mechanism is activated or encouraged by this high hormonal activity. It is important to bear in mind, however, that hormones only set the stage—*we do the rest.* There are many things we can do to offset hormonal upheavals and thereby discourage lumps and bumps from collecting in the cellulite-prone areas.

As with genetics, the best ally we can possibly have working for us is an awareness of our physiology. During pregnancy, for example, there are many precautions we can take to prevent both excessive weight gain and water retention that could otherwise become major contributing factors to a cellulite condition. This likewise holds true during periods of premenstrual syndrome (PMS), when the body tends to hold water in the hip and thigh area. Following the advice outlined in the Anti-Cellulite Strategy will greatly offset or minimize these effects.

Just as a genetic predisposition may lead us in the direction of cellulite formation, so may our hormonal makeup. Ultimately, though, neither our genes nor our hormones can be entirely to blame. The way we live has a great deal more to do with developing the actual problem than these two factors.

CELLULITE-FORMING PATTERNS

Many of the habits that later contribute to the development of cellulite become firmly established during the teen years. The lifestyle of a teenager often precludes healthy eating habits and structured physical activity. On top of this there is quite a bit of tension that arises from school, family, and peers. It is not always an easy time.

Teens often eat "on the run" or skip meals entirely. The schedule of classes and other activities is often extremely tight, leaving little time to eat decently. It is not unusual in high school for a cola and a bag of potato chips or a candy bar to serve as lunch. In college, the situation does not improve much, and cafeteria menus—notoriously heavy in salt, fats, and sugar—often provide a young student's only "real" meal. Fast food is also a major problem and one that is somewhat difficult to avoid as it is an integral part of a teenager's lifestyle.

Whether a girl learns to love or hate her body at this time can make a critical difference in the years to come. Experiments with fad diets often begin during these years when a girl is extremely sensitive to the natural changes in her body.

Studies show that two-thirds of pre–high school girls are on diets, and certain reports have yielded figures closer to 80 percent. Cycles of starving and bingeing are often established in this way—and later on may be difficult to escape. According to a study conducted at the University of Connecticut, only 20 percent of high school girls surveyed had never dieted, and 63 percent reported that they "never ate normally." It is therefore fairly obvious that a lot of imbalances, future problems, and bad habits begin right here.

Poor food choices and bad combinations put a great deal of stress on the digestive system as well as on the endocrine glands. When young, we seem to be able to get away with anything. But this abuse leads to difficulties later on.

Cellulite very often starts in the teen years but does not really "show" because of naturally taut skin and good muscle tone. Then, perhaps a decade or so later, it appears—and we wonder where it came from.

More than one cosmetic surgeon has remarked that if women took better care of themselves earlier in life—practicing good habits in nutrition and exercise—there would be far fewer patients seeking facelifts and liposuction.

Many women believe that we are somehow "programmed" to fall apart at a certain age. Yet there is rarely any thought given to the cumulative nature of this process. When we hit our thirties, somehow we just accept that this is the time to start deteriorating—it is a myth of our society, one that is generally accepted by the majority of adult women. The natural aging process is, in fact, much more subtle than that. Nature simply does not work in fits and starts.

When we're in our twenties, we tend to take things for granted, in much the same way we did as teens. We are often so busy acquiring an education, equipping ourselves with job skills, monitoring our career progress, or starting a family that we rarely take the time to care for ourselves properly. We think we will remain firm and uplifted forever. Why not? Until this time, we have been able to get away with abuse and neglect without paying any price.

Then gravity begins to take its toll, muscle tone is not quite what it should be, and the first small signs of aging appear. The experiments with various reducing diets also take their cumulative toll now. In other words, when these signs of what we call "aging" appear—including cellulite—we regard them as natural, inevitable. We fail to take into consideration that everything we've done wrong—or not done right—is now catching up with us and beginning to show.

Of course we cannot turn back the clock to adolescence and begin over again with good nutrition and regular exercise. In fact, for many of us it takes a problem like cellulite to wake us up to the abuses we've been heaping upon our bodies. Think of all the future problems you can prevent by starting right now, today, to implement good habits. And how much of the damage you can reverse.

A FINAL WORD ABOUT YOUR FIGURE... AND YOUR WEIGHT

As already stated, fat is not necessarily part of the cellulite syndrome; still, cellulite is most often present with excess fat. There are many reasons for this. Obesity, or just plain unwanted fat, is invariably caused by poor nutrition: While the body is starving for nutrients, it requires more and more food to feel satisfied. We know that poor nutrition sets off a chain reaction that leads to cellulite. Extra weight, as well as the weight regained after ineffective dieting cycles, will place a strain on the connective fibers, collagen and elastin. The eventual weakening of these fragile fibers will make cellulite more visible because of the resulting sagging or draping of skin.

Since cellulite forms in the adipose tissue, it is to our advantage to try to keep this layer to a minimum. In other words, maintaining one's proper weight is an important first step. It is now generally recognized that there is no need to add inches to our figures as we add years to our lives. The weight and shape that we reach by age twenty-five, provided these are in good proportion to our body type, should be maintained with little effort over a lifetime. Consistent weight management should be a priority. A 2- to 5-pound fluctuation, with the exception of pregnancy, is the normal range.

There are no set criteria as to what we should look like. Each of us must determine what our "ideal figure" is. This should represent, above all, a harmonious relationship between body frame and the distribution of fatty tissue that forms the lovely contours and gentle curves of the feminine body. The "perfect figure" depicted in the mass media is *not* the one to strive for. The perfect figure is our own when it is developed in natural proportion to bone structure and body type.

Obviously, we cannot change certain features, such as our height and basic frame, which are genetically programmed. What we can improve is proportion and tone. A "good body" is a healthy body, one that is tight-muscled and firm-fleshed with no extra bloating, puffiness, or padding. It is fit and glowing with vitality. This is, in fact, the way Nature intended our bodies to develop and remain over a lifetime. Careful nutrition, proper exercise, and stress management take us a long way toward achieving this goal.

4

Cellulite Reversal

A TOTAL APPROACH

Chapters 1–3 have equipped you with a great deal of information that you have no doubt already begun to think about and will soon put into practice. The remarkable beauty of this approach to cellulite reversal is the very idea of understanding basic body physiology and then working in harmony with the body, not against it. There are no gimmicks here and no flimsy promises. Your continuing success in your effort to eliminate cellulite will depend to a large degree upon how well you understand the principles we have just discussed.

It is very important to keep in mind that controlling cellulite is a way of life, that the biggest culprit in the cellulite story is *the way we live*. It makes sense, then, that some changes must be made in order to achieve lasting results. These are not radical changes in the sense of turning your life upside down, nor are they especially difficult to make. I always like to emphasize that making these changes depends so much upon our understanding of *why* we are doing so. This awareness in itself serves as a guide to keep us on the right track day after day, year after year.

The body works ceaselessly. Our trillions of cells are active twenty-four hours a day. It is up to us to cooperate with Nature in keeping the body in top condition. Paying attention to a problem for a short while and

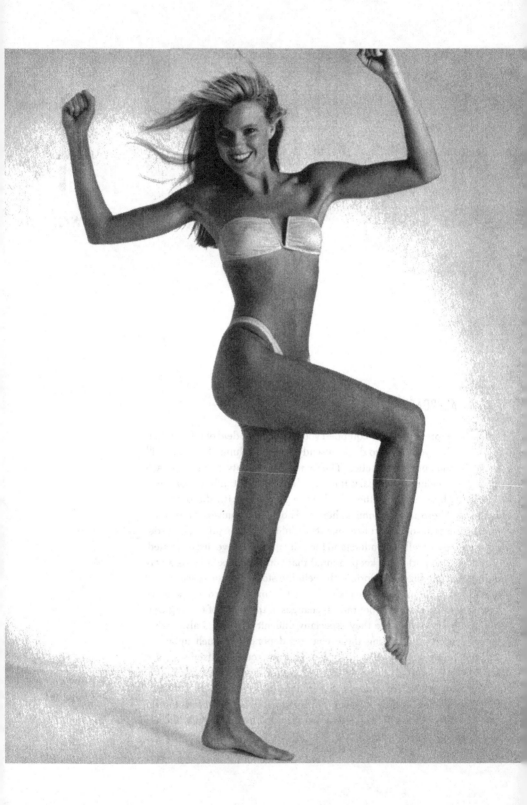

then following with complete neglect will get you nowhere. What we need is a smooth, consistent program that brings about gradual and permanent results. The effort that we put in will pay off handsomely in ways that go well beyond cellulite control.

Our immediate goal is to eliminate the unsightly and frustrating problem called cellulite. These lumps, ripples, and bulges did not appear overnight, but we still want them to disappear immediately. Try to be a little patient; and imagine that in six months to a year, your body will have improved beyond your wildest expectations.

Our ultimate goal takes us beyond cellulite. By this I mean that the results and benefits of this program are astonishingly comprehensive. As you begin to improve total body physiology with the principles of correct nutrition, targeted exercise, "skin workout," and stress management, you will notice improvement in many areas that reach far beyond the cellulite condition.

If you are conscientious and determined, you will no doubt notice results within a relatively short time—probably just a few weeks. Then the benefits accrue steadily as the natural result of the new way of life. Your overall health and sense of well-being will improve dramatically. If you currently experience certain persistent problems with digestion or elimination, these will slowly disappear. You will notice that you get fewer colds, headaches, general pains, and other low-grade health disturbances.

Premature aging will be arrested as your skin takes on a new freshness and glow. You will not tire as easily as perhaps you do now. In fact, you will have energy to spare as you glide through your work into your leisure hours. Problems that once seemed nearly insurmountable will become much easier to solve, partly because of increased vitality and partly because you will feel a greater sense of control in all phases of your life. This is certainly not a bad payoff for having made a few changes.

It is important to remember that Nature never acts quickly. While the body is remarkably resilient and extremely responsive to change, it has its own built-in timetable. It is never a good idea to interfere with this by trying to rush or force results. This is the drastic failing of diets that deprive you of essential nutrients in order to take off pounds in a hurry—and then, within a short time, you find yourself back at your prediet weight or even heavier. It is almost impossible to "trick" the body with extreme measures that attempt to circumvent its rhythms. The Anti-Cellulite Strategy takes Nature's schedule into consideration and does not violate the fundamental rules that govern physiology. Gradual improvement will bring about the kinds of results that are more likely to become permanent while keeping you in glowing health.

Remember, we are treating cellulite from the inside out, the *only* way it can be treated effectively. This means that we are treating its root cause, the disturbance at cell level that leads to congestion in the tissue spaces and the tissue damage that results. Over a period of time, the lumps will smooth out, and the bulges will diminish as muscles firm up and excess fat and fluid are eliminated. The tissue itself will become healthier and firmer. Damaged tissue will gradually be replaced with healthy tissue as cells renew and repair themselves. As we accomplish these goals, we cannot help but notice positive changes in the way we look and feel. This is the real beauty of such a total program.

Keep in mind that to be in good health means more than just being free of disease. The development of cellulite from its earliest stages indicates that there is an imbalance in the body, a problem that begins internally before it is manifested externally. By the time we see the ripples and bulges, the "internal environment" has already become congested and sluggish with the accumulation of fat, water, and wastes. This condition certainly represents something less than perfect health, and that is precisely what we seek to improve with our whole-body approach. All the interrelated systems and functions of the body will respond to the changes as we work toward optimum health and fitness.

Moderation and common sense are at the very heart of this program. What we are doing is augmenting our own best judgment with some specific guidelines that will make it easier to follow the program unerringly. Once we have managed to put the guidelines into daily practice, the rest follows naturally. Cellulite is eliminated permanently as we take control of the entire situation that brought it about.

AN OVERVIEW OF OUR PROGRAM

The Anti-Cellulite Strategy, which comprises the core of this book, focuses on four important areas: nutrition, exercise, body care, and the mind/body connection. This comprehensive plan takes into consideration total physiology as well as the changes in attitude that are necessary to banish cellulite permanently. If followed carefully, this plan will enable you to make dramatic changes in the way you look as well as in the way you feel. It is important to understand that all four phases of the plan are essential as they are designed to work together. This is the only sure way to achieve maximum results.

Eating Right

The sound and flexible eating plan emphasizes fresh, lean, nutrient-rich foods. Priority is given to complex carbohydrates—fruits, vegetables, whole grains, and legumes. These are the richest sources of potassium, the foundation of this nutritional program. These naturally thinning foods will restore the body's sodium-potassium balance while clearing up congestion in the tissue spaces. This congestive buildup is at the very root of the cellulite problem and only by dissolving and removing this tissue sludge can we make a difference in the external appearance.

These foods provide maximum nourishment as they cleanse the body of accumulated impurities and excess water. Water retention, a major contributing factor to cellulite, will be prevented through proper nourishment. There are also some suggestions for repairing damage to the skin's support system with foods that enhance collagen renewal. All the while, energy will be maintained at an exceptionally high level.

An important part of this way of eating is our very approach to food. We must cultivate a new, or at least a modified, attitude toward everything we eat. Foods must be evaluated on the basis of the nourishment they provide as well as their cleansing or purifying functions. Certain foods contribute to a cellulite condition while others help eradicate it. Once you have developed your own system for selecting the correct foods, you will be able to make the right choices with a minimum of deliberation. This new way of eating will become second nature, and you will marvel at the ease and flexibility of a plan that helps you achieve and maintain ideal weight, frees your figure of lumps and bulges, provides maximum energy, and keeps you fit and healthy.

Effective Exercise

While food builds a beautiful body, exercise shapes and sculpts it. Two types of exercise are essential in the Anti-Cellulite Strategy: those that condition the whole body and those that firm specific muscles. The former, usually called aerobics, are "low intensity" in nature and provide wonderful benefits for the cardiovascular system. By encouraging better circulation of the blood and lymph, these exercises work on the root cause of cellulite. Improved circulation will result in better distribution and assimilation of nutrients as well as more efficient removal of wastes. Many suggestions are provided for *Whole Body Conditioners*—such as walking, swimming, and bicycling—that are easily incorporated into your daily routine.

Muscle firming exercises—the *Body Shapers*—zero in to tone, tighten, lift, and remodel problem areas. These isolation-type movements are very powerful and very effective in reshaping the thighs, buttocks, waistline, and stomach. What's more, they're easy to do, take little time, and show fast results.

Breathing is a key function in our program. Not only does it bring oxygen to cells, it also controls the flow of lymph. Specific breathing exercises are provided to encourage better lymphatic circulation and maximum oxygenation of tissues. This is crucial to the elimination of cellulite. Deep breathing works wonders in raising energy levels while at the same time it cleanses the body of waste materials.

Skin Workout

Simple but effective massage techniques can greatly speed up the elimination of cellulite. Because of their stimulating action on the tissues beneath the skin, dry skin brushing and self-massage (explained later) will help smooth out lumps, improve skin tone, stimulate microcirculation, and increase lymph drainage.

The skin is a vital living organ, the body's largest, and it performs a multiplicity of functions among which is the elimination of wastes. By keeping the skin in top shape, we can greatly enhance its functioning while improving its texture and appearance.

Stress Management and Visualization

The connection between mind and body is a critical one for many reasons. Because stress is a chief contributing factor to cellulite, we must learn to control or offset its potentially devastating effects. Specific de-stressing techniques are included here to help you cope with the tensions and anxieties of daily life. Autogenic Training, in particular, works in only minutes a day to induce a state of deep relaxation. It is the ideal preparation for the visualization exercises that follow the section on stress management.

Visualization plays a key role in eliminating cellulite in many ways. With proper concentration of mental energy, we can actually enhance some of the body's functions. By imagining the way we wish to look, we can take important steps toward achieving the goal. Specific visualization techniques can help reduce lumps and bulges, improve overall physiology, hasten tissue repair, and firm the body.

PUTTING IT ALL TOGETHER

The four steps outlined above work in close harmony with one another to yield effective results. They are complementary in every way: by approaching the problem from different "directions," so to speak, we maximize our control over the body and encourage improved functioning in every area. It is the simultaneous nature of these four phases that will enable you to experience maximum improvement in the shortest possible time. With this in mind, you are ready to launch your own Anti-Cellulite Strategy, one that will dramatically and lastingly improve your figure, your overall looks, and your level of health.

Part Two THE
ANTI-CELLULITE
STRATEGY

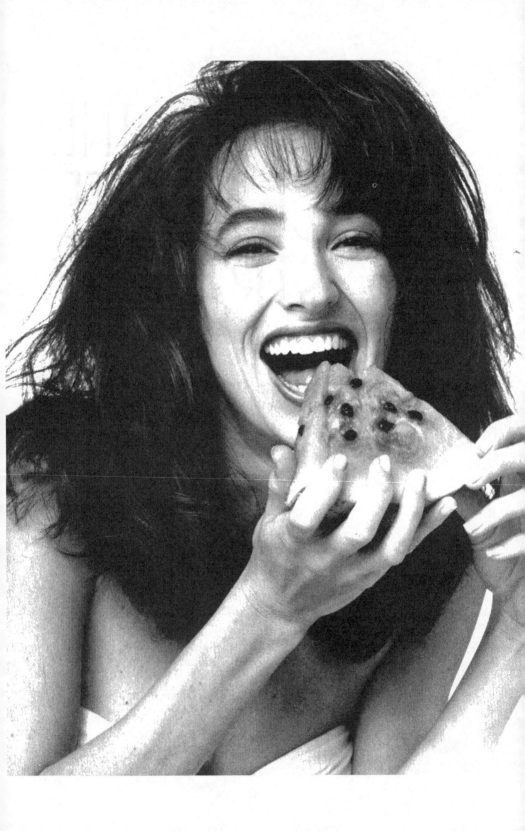

5

Eating Right

Making a commitment to "eating right" is the first step toward eliminating cellulite. Once this decision is made, a multitude of benefits follow from it—naturally, automatically, and easily. While there is no such thing as a specific "diet" that will rid you of cellulite, a sound, well-balanced eating plan that emphasizes fresh, lean, nutrient-rich foods will work wonders in dissolving the accumulation of lumps, bumps, and bulges. It's really that simple. A proper approach to nutrition sustained over a lifetime assures good health, good looks, a high level of energy, *and* a firm, trim body free of ripples and distorting bulges.

I've never believed in dieting in the conventional sense. This implies not only a temporary state of denial and deprivation but leads to nutritional imbalances and deficiencies. No good can be derived from this kind of program—mentally or physically. A diet should really be called "the right way to eat." Do not even consider going on a diet that you couldn't live with for the rest of your life. A diet is not something you "go on" for a few weeks or a few months. It's a way to eat—forever.

I have always believed that the correct way of feeding the body means plenty of good food in the right proportions and combinations. There are no mysteries here, but for many this may require undoing certain bad habits and replacing them with good ones. The changes should be gradual, as the mind and body adjust to accommodate a new set of behaviors.

A proper diet includes carbohydrates, protein, and fat in the correct ratio and from the right sources. It is the proper balance of these three that maintains a healthy, slim, well-functioning body. Such a diet emphasizes fresh foods—high in potassium, water content, and fiber—and very little, if any, processed foods. It is low in fat, salt, sugar, caffeine, and alcohol.

Most people do not eat properly. Despite all the awareness about nutrition that has developed in recent years, statistics show that the average person still eats about twice the amount of required protein, four to five times the amount of fat necessary for the body's needs, ten to fifteen times the sodium needed, and nearly a third of a pound of sugar a day. A lot of this is due to the fact that the average diet relies heavily on processed foods and includes too many sweets, salty snacks, and sugary drinks. Over half the calories supplied by such a diet are totally devoid of nutrients. This way of eating results in low energy, extreme blood sugar variations, excess weight, cellulite, and a host of subhealth conditions.

Learning to eat properly, first of all, means learning to distinguish the foods that provide essential nutrients. The foods that best sustain the human body with maximum nourishment and minimum waste are the complex carbohydrates. These foods—vegetables, fruits, whole grains, and legumes such as peas, beans, and lentils—are given priority in our sound and flexible eating plan. They are also the richest sources of potassium, our secret weapon in fighting cellulite.

Potassium-rich foods restore the optimal sodium-potassium ratio and water balance in the body. They raise the energy potential of cells and thus render them more efficient at picking up nutrients and expelling waste products. They also eliminate and/or prevent water retention and flush out excess salt stored in tissues.

Complex carbohydrates are truly in harmony with the body. They are the safest foods for our health, the only ones not associated with degenerative diseases and premature aging. And they do have a track record that goes back thousands of years. They are the "clean fuel" of the body, leaving only water and carbon dioxide as end products, which the body can easily dispose of, unlike animal foods—meat, dairy products, and so forth—which leave an enormous amount of waste and put extra strain on the body for their elimination.

Complex carbohydrates are naturally thinning foods and should make up the largest portion of your diet. They provide high bulk and have a high satiety value. Because they are absorbed slowly into the system, they keep your blood sugar stable and your energy high. They are also naturally low in fat—an important consideration for an efficient, easy-flowing circulation and the vital transport of oxygen, nutrients, enzymes, and hormones to individual cells. Less dietary fat also means less body fat. Part of the beauty of this eating plan is that it allows for weight loss for those who need it while others easily maintain ideal weight.

Food is meant to cleanse the body as it nourishes. When we accomplish this dual purpose, we are really getting the maximum benefit from what we eat rather than simply eating to satisfy the appetite. This cleansing function is vital to health and crucial to banishing cellulite. The congestive buildup of "tissue sludge" that characterizes cellulite is broken down as we systematically perform this cleansing function at cell level. This is the only way to reestablish order in the internal environment where the problem resides. Fruits, vegetables, salads, and sprouts, most of them in their raw state—high in potassium, enzymes, fiber, and water—gradually detoxify the system.

Water is the ultimate purifier of the body, the total cleanser that keeps everything flowing and in balance. Besides eating foods that are naturally high in water content, drinking plenty of water in the right ways and at the right times will further assure adequate hydration and gradual detoxification.

There is a certain amount of tissue damage that takes place with cellulite buildup. We can repair much of this damage with foods that restore collagen and elastin fibers to a healthier state. This is exceedingly important in maintaining the firm, healthy appearance of surface skin. The congestion that forms to create cellulite in the first place "chokes" this tissue, giving it a dull, devitalized look. As cells repair and renew themselves, amazing changes begin to take place within the tissue and lead directly to dramatic improvements in appearance—firmer, fresher, younger-looking skin.

Good digestion is *key* in this program. When foods are not digested properly, nutrients cannot be assimilated—and assimilation is really the name of the game in nutrition. No matter how good your diet, if nutrients are not absorbed you will reap no benefit. What really counts is not only how much we eat but how much we absorb and utilize. Thus, proper eating habits—*how* we eat—is just as important as *what* we eat.

DIETING MAKES YOU FAT... AND FLABBY

The whole concept of dieting is generally negative. Rarely is there a focus on nourishing the body with good, wholesome, nutrient-rich foods. And so, most diets yield results that are counterproductive in the end.

Usually a diet is regarded as an extreme measure to take off weight for a special event, for a vacation, or to fit into last year's bathing suit without any extra bulges as evidence of neglect. Such dieting often leads to postdiet bingeing simply because of the deprivation that has been endured. What's more, the weight that is lost almost always comes back—in many cases, with a few extra pounds. The failure rate following crash diets is 90 percent. Thus, the cycle is self-perpetuating.

There are several reasons why diets fail. In addition to the psychological implications of temporary deprivation, these diets generally leave little energy or incentive for exercise. When dieting is not accompanied by exercise, the body responds with a slower metabolism to accommodate the reduced caloric intake. This leads to increased difficulty in further weight loss.

When you lose weight too rapidly, muscle tissue is sacrificed in the process. While you achieve a slimmer silhouette, you are left fatter "inside." Repeated dieting will only make matters worse because you are simply decreasing more muscle and adding more fat.

Losing weight properly means learning to eat correctly and to exercise regularly. This balanced equation of nutrition and exercise is really the only way to achieve your ideal weight and to maintain it permanently. Keep in mind that your ideal weight is one that you can easily maintain without unnecessary starvation and loss of energy. If you have to starve yourself to maintain a certain weight, your body is telling you that this is not the right weight for you. The rate of weight loss should not exceed one pound per week—this way, you should be able to lose stored fat without losing muscle tissue.

TISSUE DAMAGE... ANOTHER CONSEQUENCE OF DIETING

As subcutaneous tissue increases in volume, you are increasing your chances of developing cellulite in the areas where the body naturally stores fat: hips, thighs, buttocks, and stomach. Also, as the skin in these areas stretches and restretches to accommodate the variations in volume, damage occurs to the underlying support network. The delicate collagen and elastin fibers can handle only so much stretching before they are weakened and lose elasticity. As we get older, this stretching becomes more critical. Furthermore, dieting robs your skin of precious collagen by depriving the body of the very nutrients that enhance collagen renewal.

In many instances, women specifically undertake drastic dieting to lose cellulite. When the expected results do not occur, they diet even more. Now, the all-too-famous trio is set into motion: deprivation-frustration-bingeing. The accompanying loss of muscle tissue will actually leave more room for cellulite to form and spread. And the damage that is done to connective tissue will allow this process to continue with increasingly visible results.

The bottom line is: Don't diet. . . . Eat right all the time.

The right foods, the ones that feed the body, can be eaten in plenty. Fresh fruits, fresh vegetables, whole grains, and legumes provide a great amount of bulk, which satisfies the appetite quickly and is easily digested and assimilated. These foods will prevent the loss of vital muscle tissue as they encourage the loss of unwanted fat.

WHAT ABOUT CALORIES?

All calories are not equal. It's really a question of quality versus quantity. Calories from fat are the ones you need to worry about: They are the most fattening. One of the reasons for this is the ease with which the body converts dietary fat into body fat. The process of digestion itself actually burns calories—for fat, only about 3 percent; for complex carbohydrates the output of digestive energy is significantly higher, about 23 percent. This is why "fat" calories—97 percent of them—are stored as body fat.

So the next time you look at calorie charts, check out the sources of those calories and go for the "lean" type. Try to think of foods this way: "firm" foods, such as vegetables and whole grains, will make firm tissue; "fatty" foods, such as butter, cheese, and meat, will make fatty tissue.

Also bear in mind that activity has a great deal to do with how many calories are needed by your body. This varies with your expenditure of energy—and energy needs vary enormously among individuals. For most people, the daily food intake should not drop below 1,200–1,300 calories. This is the minimum you will need if you are to exercise effectively, a must in any health-sustaining program, and it's the minimum that allows you to get all the nutrients you need including vitamins and minerals.

EATING RIGHT... AT A GLANCE

To get lasting results you must remove the cause not just the symptoms. In other words, bring the body into a state of balance. The first thing you need to do will be to stop putting in your body the substances you know are not good for you. The second step will be to start giving your body the essential nutrients it needs.

Cut out as much as possible:

    —Processed food

Cut down on:

    —Meat
    —Dairy products
    —Fats
    —Sugar
    —Salt

THE ANTI-CELLULITE WAY TO EAT

Emphasize fresh, lean, nutrient-rich foods. Give priority to the complex carbohydrates:

—Fruits
—Vegetables
—Whole grains
—Legumes

These foods are the richest sources of potassium, the foundation of our eating plan. A substantial portion of fruits and vegetables should be eaten raw since raw foods are an integral part of this program.

In addition, drink plenty of pure water, six to eight glasses a day.

This plan will:

—Restore optimal sodium-potassium balance in tissues
—Correct nutritional deficiencies that lead to cellulite
—Clear up congestion in tissue spaces
—Nourish and cleanse the body
—Heal and repair tissues
—Prevent or eliminate water retention
—Promote weight loss—if needed
—Maintain ideal weight effortlessly
—Keep energy level high

CUT OUT AS MUCH PROCESSED FOOD AS POSSIBLE

This is a major step in your diet, and it is first on the list of things to avoid for good reasons. Processed foods are the number-one troublemakers in our so-called modern diet of refined, convenient, altered substances that barely resemble food. Most are loaded with huge amounts of salt, fat, and sugar plus loads of chemicals our bodies have no use for. In addition to these negatives, most nutrients are either lost completely or greatly diminished in processing. While we are being offered "enriched" or "fortified" foods, what we get is close to nothing in terms of nutrients and a lot more than we bargained for in terms of undesirable ingredients.

There are over two thousand chemical additives used in the food industry. Many of these have not been tested adequately and none have been tested in combination with one another. Thousands more find their way into our food as it is grown, processed, packaged, and stored, and there are no federal regulations requiring them to be listed on labels. These chemicals include hormones and antibiotics fed to animals, pesticides sprayed on plants and crops, and residues from substances used to clean equipment. Our bodies are not equipped to deal with so many chemicals, many of which are stored in our organs and tissues, often in adipose tissue.

In 1960, the average American consumed 2 pounds of chemical additives in food. By 1978, this increased to 10 pounds. We can only guess what the consumption is by now. Our first defense is to read labels carefully. Not all food additives are necessarily bad—many are used for our protection. But do we need thousands? Be your own judge.

Food is meant to nourish, repair, and strengthen the trillions of cells in our bodies. In order to function, we need nutrients. Considering that processed foods constitute the largest part of the diet for the majority of people, it's astonishing that we function at all. This is not to mention that processed junk food is the major cause of obesity in our society and is associated with most degenerative diseases. What is wrong with the food we eat is not always its quantity but its lack of quality.

Processed foods are a form of manipulation. Examine your own eating habits carefully. Shouldn't *you* control how much fat, sugar, and salt goes into your body? Shouldn't *you* decide how many chemicals you want to risk your health on?

Fresh food is always better than processed. The more a food has been tampered with, the less nourishing it is. The closer a food is to its natural state, the more nourishing it is. When shopping, put emphasis on whole, fresh foods and not those that are fragmented, altered, and devitalized. Try to deemphasize or eliminate processed foods, fast foods, and junk foods. Keep in mind that the longer the shelf life of a product, the higher its levels of fat, salt, and chemicals.

Once you cut out processed foods and cut down on meat—our next step—you're halfway home nutritionally. The benefits are, literally, immediate.

CUT DOWN ON MEAT

Meat—red meat especially—is very high in fat calories—even the so-called lean cuts. What's more, most meats contain a variety of chemicals, antibiotics, synthetic hormones, and pesticide residues. Many of these chemicals collect in the liver of the animal—a good reason to cut down on this popular organ meat.

Cold cuts especially are loaded with a multitude of undesirable chemicals besides being extremely high in salt. Try to avoid all cold cuts from the deli counter as well as the packaged varieties. If you look carefully in your own neighborhood, more than likely you'll find a delicatessen that prepares its own turkey and roast beef without the additives.

As for poultry, try to choose the leanest varieties. They are less "yellow" in appearance—for example, fryers have less fat than roasters. Turkey is quite lean.

In general, try to shift your emphasis away from meat to other sources of protein. When possible, try to substitute fish for meat. But if you continue to include meat in your diet, here are some useful guidelines:

- Try to eat meat no more than twice a week.
- Choose the leanest possible cuts and trim all visible fat.
- Use meat more as a garnish or flavoring than as a main course.
- Prepare meats either by broiling or poaching rather than frying.

CUT DOWN ON DAIRY PRODUCTS

Dairy products are the traditional source of calcium and a major source of protein. Yet at the same time, many of them are rich in fats—especially cheese, which also happens to be high in salt. Therefore, you must select carefully and consume dairy products judiciously.

Bear in mind also that dairy products are not the only sources of calcium. All green vegetables are very rich in this mineral: broccoli, kale, spinach, and watercress as well as beet, collard, and turnip greens. Parsley and sprouts are also rich sources, as are carrots. Other sources are nuts, seeds, tofu, whole-grain breads, and cereals.

As for Yogurt

The best choice is plain low-fat yogurt. You can add your own sweetener in the form of fresh fruit, currants (these are lower in calories than raisins and higher in fiber), or even a teaspoon of "fruit only" preserves (with no sugar added).

Cheese

Low-fat cheeses are your best choice: cottage cheese, part-skim mozzarella, and part-skim ricotta. Medium-fat cheeses are Neufchâtel, Swiss, and Parmesan. Freshly grated Parmesan can add a zesty flavor to many foods but very little is needed—try to sprinkle rather than pour as it's extremely high in salt. In general, most hard cheeses are high in fat and should be eaten with discretion. You will be likely to use less if you grate it or slice it with a cheese parer that skims off thin slivers.

An excellent way of indulging your taste for cheese is to grate or cube a very small amount into a salad as a garnish. As a general rule, try not to consume more than 1 or 2 ounces of cheese at a time and not more than three times a week.

Milk

Use only low-fat or skimmed.

WHAT ABOUT PROTEIN?

We need this essential nutrient to build and repair tissues, which is, in fact, its main function. Indeed, every cell in your body contains some protein. But even though protein plays such an important role, you don't need very much. The key here again is **quality** not **quantity**.

Most people consume two to three times the amount of protein they need, primarily from animal sources. Too much protein depletes the body of essential minerals, including potassium, and creates an inordinate amount of toxic waste, the natural by-product of protein metabolism. This puts extra strain on the kidneys, which are forced to work overtime to excrete these wastes.

Contrary to popular belief, protein does not "build" muscle directly—it requires the presence of carbohydrates—it is not an efficient source of energy, and it does not have magical powers to assist in weight reduction.

Generally, you need not be concerned about getting too little protein. If you eat properly, the need for protein can be met without much calculation. A diet centered around vegetables, whole grains, and legumes will provide you with all you need.

Protein is everywhere. The best strategy is to obtain most of your protein from plant sources. Think of animal protein—meats and dairy products—as the garnish or flavoring to your meal rather than the centerpiece.

Cut Down on Fats

Fat, not surprisingly, is our most fattening nutrient, and it is the one we need in the least amount. After all, less fat in your diet means less fat on your body. Not only do fats make us fat, they also clog circulation and add to the burden of damaging free radicals in the system.

While it is true that carbohydrates, protein, and fat are essential to a healthy, balanced diet, they are not required in equal proportions. The ideal diet for optimal nutrition should consist of 60–70 percent complex carbohydrates, 10–15 percent protein, and 15–20 percent fat. Compare this with the average American diet, which is bountiful but hardly balanced: 40 percent carbohydrates (mostly from simple carbohydrates such as sugar and refined flour), 25 percent protein, and an astounding 45–50 percent fat. It's quite obvious that most people would benefit enormously by increasing carbohydrate intake (from the right sources), decreasing protein, and drastically curtailing fats. They would be a lot slimmer, too.

You may not think you eat a lot of fat, but chances are you're eating much more than you realize. This is because most of the fat we consume comes to us from "hidden" sources. In some cases it is a natural part of the food, such as with meat and cheese. In other cases it is added during preparation—cream and butter-based sauces, french fries, and so on. Of course, a tremendous amount of fat is added to processed and fast foods.

Many nutritious low-calorie, low-fat foods are transformed into fat-laden ones by the way they are prepared or served. The potato is a good example: In its natural state, 8 ounces of potatoes has only 2 calories that come from fat. If you fry the same amount of potatoes, you add 220 fat calories! Pasta is another typical example: By itself, it is naturally low in fat. When it is dished up with gobs of sauce, especially the cream varieties, it becomes outrageously fattening.

There are many simple ways to curtail fat intake, sometimes drastically. Here are a few tips to "de-fat" your diet:

- Always use nonstick pots and pans that will allow you to use a minimum of fat or none at all.
- Use only a touch of butter or just a bit of oil when needed. Or use a nonstick vegetable oil spray.
- Use whipped butter rather than regular butter. It has substantially less fat. Margarine is not necessarily a better choice healthwise. Better have the real thing but less of it. Moderation in all things is the best way to go. Also, substitute vegetable oil whenever possible, in baking for example.
- Use a squeeze of fresh lemon on cooked vegetables rather than a chunk of butter or margarine. A few drops of oil or a dash of freshly grated Parmesan cheese will also add delicious flavor.
- Whenever possible, substitute plain yogurt for sour cream, but if you must use sour cream, look for the low-fat variety.
- When buying canned tuna, sardines, and salmon, select only the water-packed varieties.
- If you must use cream cheese occasionally—and many have a weakness for it, especially on a bagel—stick to the whipped variety as it has a third less fat. And spread it thin—no globs.
- Use mayonnaise sparingly—never drown or saturate foods with it. Whenever possible, look for a reduced-calorie, low-sodium brand. A good way to stretch mayonnaise is by using half plain yogurt.
- Replace half the oil in your salad dressing with plain yogurt or puréed cucumber.

What About the Fat We Need?

Eating some fat is essential to health, but as you will see, very little of it is needed. Fat is necessary to the formation of delicate cell membranes as well as the synthesis of hormones. It is required for the transport and absorption of the fat-soluble vitamins A, D, E, and K. Also, fat keeps your skin and other tissues youthful by preventing dryness and scaliness.

The body's daily requirements for essential fatty acids—those that the body cannot make on its own—can be met with a mere tablespoon or two (3 to 6 teaspoons) of polyunsaturated fats. No more than 10–20 percent of your total calories should come from fat. A high fat intake can only spell trouble for one's health as well as one's weight. The real key to using fats is small amounts.

Watch Out for Heated Fats

By all means, avoid deep-fried foods: french fries, onion rings, fried fish, potato chips, doughnuts, and the like. When fats are heated to high temperatures the chemical structure changes. Thus altered, fat becomes totally indigestible, even toxic. This is one good reason why you should never reheat oils already used. It is also why commercially fried foods should be avoided completely. The fats used in restaurants, for example, are used over and over—they are totally polluted.

When you stir-fry at home, use only the smallest amount of oil and *never* heat to the smoking point. Olive, peanut, and sesame oils are particularly suitable for this purpose.

Vegetable Oils

Commercial oils are extracted with the aid of chemical solvents and are heated at extremely high temperatures. The final product here is degenerated and completely stripped of any valuable nutrients.

Look for oils that specify how they were extracted. These will bear the expressions "cold pressed," "unrefined," or "extra virgin" on their labels. Buy oils in small containers and keep them refrigerated (except for olive oil, which keeps for a long while at room temperature). Otherwise, they can easily turn rancid and thus release dangerous free radicals.

Cut Down on Sugar

Despite all that has been written and said about the deleterious effects of sugar—from mood swings to diabetes, hypoglycemia, lowered immunity, obesity, and tooth decay—the average American is now consuming around 130 pounds per year. This is 2½ pounds per week! Our bodies have absolutely no physiological need for refined sugar. Moreover, sugar depletes the body of precious potassium—one more reason to stay away from the stuff.

Most of this sugar comes to us in "hidden" forms. Because of this, even people who claim not to eat sweets consume far more sugar than they realize. Sugar is the number-one additive in foods. It is used in practically everything from ketchup and other condiments to bread, crackers, nondairy creamers, cured meats, salad dressings, spaghetti sauce, and bouillon cubes—to name just a few common items. This is not to mention the obvious sources, such as soft drinks, cookies, ice cream, and candy. Sugar, like salt, is an acquired taste. And it brings you nothing at all except empty calories and a craving for more.

Sugar by any other name—fructose, brown sugar, raw sugar—is still sugar. Honey, molasses, and maple syrup may provide a few minerals, but they are also sugar and must be used in moderation. This is not to say that we should never use sugar. This would be unrealistic. However, when a sweetener is called for, use it sparingly.

Artificial sweeteners don't do much besides perpetuate your taste for sweets. They should be used only as a "crutch" while you decrease your sugar intake. None of these products is totally safe. The best advice for using artificial sweeteners is to use them if you must but in moderation.

Here are a few tips to help you cut down your sugar intake and lose your taste for unneeded sweets:

- First and foremost, try to stay away from processed foods as much as possible. The more you cut down on these, the more you will curb your taste for sweets—and the less sugar your body will have to convert into fat.
- When cooking or baking at home, reduce the amount of sugar in recipes by half. You'll be surprised how this will not affect the finished product—and you'll be way ahead. After a while, you can cut down even more.
- If you're hungry for something sweet, reach for fresh fruit. Always buy fruit that's in season, since it usually tastes much better—and no matter what the season, there is always some fruit available.
- Avoid canned fruit. If you must use it from time to time, only buy the kind packed in its own juice.
- Read labels carefully on the processed foods that you must buy. If sugar is listed among the first ingredients, you're in trouble. If it comes last, don't worry too much. Little by little, you'll learn to substitute other products with less or no sugar added. After a while, you'll find that overly sweet foods make you feel nauseated.
- Buy "fruit only" preserves without any added sugar. These are widely available in health food stores as well as supermarkets. You can also make your own fruit purée by processing very ripe fruit in the blender.
- Do not keep in the house anything that you don't want to eat or drink, such as ice cream, candy, cookies, soft drinks. If you don't have these things, you won't be tempted.
- If you use sugar in your coffee or tea, gradually reduce the amount. Before long, you'll be able to give it up completely.

Cut Down on Salt

Most of us eat far too much salt—on average, more than twenty times what the body needs. Yes, it is true that we need sodium to remain healthy: It regulates cellular fluid pressure, controls pH balance in the body, and maintains calcium suspension in the bloodstream. Yet all the salt we need is contained in nearly every food we eat. And that's exactly how we should consume it: as it occurs naturally in foods. The salt we add to foods while cooking and at the table, and the salt added to processed foods, is the salt that spells danger.

While we need not worry about getting too little salt, most of us ought to worry about getting too much. Sodium accounts for about 2 percent of the body's mineral content, and that small percentage is important. It is present mainly in the fluid that surrounds cells, and when it is properly balanced with potassium, it speeds nutrients into cells and waste products out. Remember, this delicate balance of sodium and potassium is largely responsible for maintaining a clean, healthy internal environment. Too much sodium in the body will interfere with fluid balance: Salt retains approximately seventy times its weight in water.

To remember how mineral concentration affects fluid volume, keep in mind this short sentence: Where sodium goes, water soon follows. Too much salt results in potassium deficiency and water retention, which causes bloating and accentuates cellulite.

Aside from its effect on water retention, cell metabolism, and the formation of cellulite, salt is definitely detrimental to our health. It is a form of poison to the body, just like sugar. And, as with sugar, the taste for salt is an acquired one that can be broken fairly easily. This does not mean that we must live the rest of our lives on a salt-free diet—unless medically required—but most of us should seriously consider cutting down drastically. Contrary to what most people think, salt does not enhance the taste of foods, it masks it.

Our daily sodium intake, according to the National Academy of Sciences, should be between 1,000 and 3,300 milligrams from all sources. This amounts to ½–1½ teaspoons. The minimum requirement is actually very low: only 200 milligrams a day. A breakfast of two fried eggs, two strips of bacon, and a single slice of whole wheat toast contains nearly 1,100 milligrams of sodium—and that's without adding any table salt. One pickle alone contains 934 milligrams. This gives you an idea of how far we exceed the minimum and the recommended intake. And some of us do that by lunchtime!

It has been estimated that the average American gets about 15 percent of his sodium from the salt shaker, another 10 percent occurs in foods naturally. The remaining 75 percent comes from processed foods—and this portion is even higher for those who eat frequently in restaurants. The many thousands of high-sodium processed foods contain dangerous levels of hidden salt. And most antacids and many over-the-counter medications also have very high sodium contents.

As with all dietary changes, reducing salt should be accomplished gradually. You will be less likely to notice the difference, more likely to adapt easily, and far more likely to make the reduced intake a habit if you cut down little by little. Before you know it, you'll be down to a mere fraction of the amount you once used. And you will never miss the salt because your taste buds will have a chance to "wake up" to the wonderful flavors of real foods.

Some tips for cutting down on salt include:

- Avoid commercially prepared foods that are obviously salty. Some of these, such as canned soups, contain the equivalent of an entire day's sodium supply in a single serving. Therefore, you should eliminate as much processed food as possible from your life. Canned, frozen, packaged, ready-mixed foods should be carefully avoided. With a little planning, you can prepare delicious, wholesome meals that will nourish rather than poison your body.
- Cook from "scratch" as much as possible. When you do this, you control how much salt (as well as sugar and fats) gets into your foods.
- Do not add salt when cooking. If you must add salt at all, do it on the plate after the food is prepared—and sprinkle as little as possible *after* you've tasted it. Since it will "sit" on your food instead of being in your food, you will find that you use considerably less.
- Consider switching to Morton's Lite salt, which is readily available in supermarkets. It's a mixture of half sodium and half potassium chloride. However, do not use salt substitutes made entirely of potassium chloride without your physician's advice.
- Explore the wide range of herbs and spices to enhance the flavors of foods. Garlic, pepper, and onions will add variety to your salt-reduced foods. A fresh squeeze of lemon or lime juice will also really perk up a meal. Avoid the "salty" seasonings such as garlic salt, onion salt, celery salt, seasoned salt, bouillon cubes, and steak sauce. Try wine or sherry for a sophisticated touch. Don't worry about the alcohol content; it evaporates during cooking.
- Rinse certain processed foods under running water for one minute to eliminate much of the added salt. In this manner, you can substan-

tially reduce the sodium content of such items as water-packed tuna, kidney beans, and chick-peas.

- When you buy soy sauce, try to get the reduced-sodium variety at a health food store or the health food section of a supermarket. It's often called tamari. Or make your own reduced-sodium variety by diluting tamari half and half with water. Never buy the American version of soy sauce found in supermarkets—it's far too high in sodium.
- Try low-sodium baking powder if you bake a lot. It's available in health food stores and some supermarkets.
- Read labels carefully: Any ingredient with the word *sodium* means salt. It is not unusual to see several such ingredients listed on a single item. Monosodium glutamate, sodium benzoate, sodium bicarbonate, sodium sulfite, sodium hydroxide, sodium cyclamate, sodium alginate, and sodium propionate are some of the sodium compounds you may see listed.

ALL-IMPORTANT POTASSIUM

Potassium, as mentioned, is the foundation of our eating plan. Think of this valuable mineral as the "secret weapon" in the fight against cellulite, because it is exactly that.

As explained in Chapter 2, our trillions of cells require sufficient potassium in order to function efficiently. For cells to take in oxygen and nutrients; expel wastes; repair, renew, and ultimately replace themselves—all vital to a smooth body—the proper amount of potassium must be present. When these functions do not occur at a steady and healthy pace, one of the results is the congestive buildup of cellulite. The situation compounds itself: This buildup further slows cellular activity, and the evacuation of wastes becomes more and more difficult. This disturbance in body chemistry is the crux of the cellulite problem.

Sodium and potassium, the mineral partners, work in close tandem, and they must be present in the proper ratio at all times. A lack of potassium, often caused by an excess of sodium in the diet, results in fluid retention, flabbiness, poor intestinal tone, fatigue, and muscle weakness.

Water retention, with its accompanying bloating and puffiness, can be eliminated entirely—or at least kept in check—with potassium-rich foods. Since sodium is the culprit in attracting water to tissues, by cutting way down on salt intake and loading up on potassium, you can flush out excess water stored in the body. Just this one step will make a dramatic difference in overall smoothness and firmness. Waterlogged tissue is spongy tissue. No matter how good your muscle tone, with a spongy and uneven layer of subcutaneous tissue padding those muscles, you cannot achieve a taut, sinewy appearance.

Firm, healthy tissue depends upon the efficient nourishment of every single cell that makes up that tissue. If valuable nutrients cannot reach the cells as a result of too much buildup in the tiny spaces between cells, then they are wasted. Potassium is the mineral that assures the speedy, unimpeded transport of these nutrients.

The quality of lymph depends to some degree upon potassium. Clean, evenly flowing lymph is vital to a smooth, healthy body. We can boost lymphatic circulation with exercise, of course, but if the lymphatic fluid itself is too thick and viscous—often a result of too much sodium along with trapped cellular wastes in tissue spaces—then its flow will be sluggish. Adequate potassium assures good clean lymph, which flows more evenly to cleanse the body of wastes and other impurities.

Besides its effect on cellulite, potassium is required for normal growth, muscle contraction, pH balance, healthy skin, the synthesis of protein, proper heart function, clear mental focus, and a calm disposition. For all its many health benefits, not enough attention is being given to this vital, multipurpose mineral. Surveys show that the average American consumes far too few fresh fruits and vegetables—and still far too much salt.

The first step in balancing the mineral equation is to *cut down on salt*. The next step is to *increase potassium*. The best sources of potassium are plant foods: fresh fruits, fresh vegetables, sprouts, legumes, and whole grains—the basis of our healthy eating plan. For optimum benefits, you should eat high-potassium foods throughout the day. All fruits and most vegetables contain ten to one hundred times more potassium than sodium. So it is easy to understand the importance of emphasizing these valuable foods.

In a healthy diet, the ratio of potassium to sodium should be at minimum two to one to reflect their respective proportions in the body: Potassium accounts for approximately 5 percent of the body's total mineral content, while sodium is closer to 2 percent. In other words, we should take in at the very least twice as much potassium as we do sodium. This is hardly the norm. In the average diet, sodium intake far outweighs that of potassium. Following are some typical menus that clearly illustrate this point.

	SODIUM/mg	POTASSIUM/mg
Breakfast		
Cheese omelette (2 eggs, 2 oz. American processed cheese)	922	262
Two pieces of toast	246	80
Mid-morning		
One Danish pastry	238	72
Lunch		
New England clam chowder (cup)	914	146
Chicken club sandwich	813	365
One pickle (large)	934	130

	SODIUM/mg	POTASSIUM/mg
Dinner		
Tossed salad (iceberg lettuce with creamy Italian dressing (2 tbsp.)	268	110
Lasagne with meat sauce (8 oz.) (frozen)	1000	340
Two dinner rolls	140	20
TOTALS:	5475	1525

Some common snack items are also shockingly weighted in favor of sodium.

	SODIUM/mg	POTASSIUM/mg
Pretzels, 3½ oz.	1,680	130
Saltines, 3½ oz.	1,100	120
Cheddar cheese, 3½ oz.	700	82
Green olives (10)	1,400	45
Chocolate chip cookies, 3½ oz.	1,819	608

Now, compare with some fresh fruits and vegetables:

	SODIUM/mg	POTASSIUM/mg
Acorn squash, ½ cup, baked	4	446
Artichoke, 1 medium	79	316
Avocado, ½	10	550
Banana, 1 medium	1	451
Broccoli, ½ cup	8	124
Brussels sprouts, ½ cup	17	247
Cantaloupe, ½	23	825
Carrot, 1 medium, raw	25	233
Cherries, 20	0	304
Cucumber, ½	3	250
Grapefruit, ½	0	175
Kiwi, 1	4	252
Mango, 1	4	322
Nectarine, 1	0	288
Orange, 1	0	237
Papaya, 1	8	780
Pineapple, 1 cup pieces	1	175
Potato, 1, baked with skin	16	844
Spinach, 1 cup, raw	44	312
Tomato, 1 raw	10	254
Watermelon, 1 wedge (4 × 8 in.)	2	600

Some tips for seeking out the best sources of potassium and for increasing your daily intake include:

- Oranges, bananas, and baked potatoes are the "old reliables" for high potassium. Include them regularly in your diet.
- Cantaloupe, generally available year-round, is another excellent source. Have it often. For variety, put it through a juicer or a blender—it's quite delicious.
- Watermelon is very high in potassium. Take advantage of the seasonal abundance and eat plenty. Again, for a refreshing change, try juicing or blending it—rind and all.
- Legumes such as navy beans, kidney beans, lima beans, and lentils contain lots of potassium—protein as well. All make delectable soups.
- Add potassium to your homemade soups with parsnips, rutabaga, potatoes, and acorn squash.
- Always add a shredded carrot to your salads and sandwiches for extra potassium.
- Avocados are very high in potassium and make a nice addition to salads and sandwiches. They also contain high-quality protein and essential fatty acids.
- Freshly extracted vegetable juices are a delicious way to obtain loads of potassium. For example, one cup of carrot juice contains nearly 800 mg.
- You can toss an assortment of fresh fruit into the blender for a high-potassium breakfast, appetizer, or snack. This luscious purée is unsurpassed as a refreshing potassium "cocktail."
- Preserve the high potassium content of vegetables by steaming or cooking them in as little water as possible. Homemade vegetable soup is a simple and superb way of obtaining potassium because no liquid is discarded.
- Always eat fruits and vegetables fresh. The potassium that is lost in canning and freezing is just another good reason to avoid these completely. For example, 100 grams (3½ oz.) of fresh peas contain 1 mg of sodium and 380 mg of potassium; the same amount of canned peas (drained) contains 350 mg of sodium and 180 mg of potassium. Thus, the canned product contains 350 times more sodium than fresh peas—and more than half the potassium has been lost.
- Potassium should always be taken in natural form—that is, the way it occurs naturally in foods. Avoid the pill form; it can be irritating to the digestive tract and dangerous if taken in large amounts.

FRUITS AND VEGETABLES

Think of these as your best allies. Though they are not the only foods you need, they should take centerstage in your eating plan. Both fruits and vegetables have what is called "high nutrient density," which means they contain very large amounts of essential vitamins and minerals for very few calories. What's more, they are naturally high in water content, dietary fiber, and potassium—all essential components in the fight against cellulite.

You should have three to five servings of fruits and four to six servings of vegetables daily. This can easily be accomplished as you will see in Meal Planning Ideas. For example, one or two glasses of freshly extracted fruit or vegetable juice will allow you to include a number of these items as will one or two salads per day.

Here are some useful guidelines for your consumption of fruits and vegetables:

- As a rule, it is best to shop for fresh produce often. Look for fresh, crisp varieties. Avoid those with bruises or soft spots.
- Buy no more produce than you will be able to consume in a few days.
- To preserve nutrients, store produce in a cool, dry place.
- Do not peel or cut fruits and vegetables until just prior to eating.
- Fruits and vegetables should never be soaked; instead, wash and scrub them thoroughly under cool running water.
- Cook vegetables until they are tender but still firm. Steaming and stir-frying are the best methods of preparation.
- Fruits should always be eaten raw. They make perfect snacks and appetizers.
- Always buy fruits and vegetables in season. They are at their peak of tastiness.
- Always eat fruits ripe.

THE IMPORTANCE OF RAW FOODS

Foods are most nourishing when they are as close to their natural state as possible. The more processed or devitalized a food is, the less nourishing. Fruits and vegetables are most nourishing when eaten raw—sprouted grains and legumes along with raw nuts and seeds provide excellent sources of whole nutrition.

Raw foods are vital to optimum health and energy levels—and invaluable in fighting cellulite. Real nutrition means "feeding" our trillions of cells—enabling them to repair, replenish, and replace themselves efficiently—and cleansing the body of wastes. True, we are sustained even when we eat foods that don't do that—namely processed foods, refined foods, and cooked foods—but our cells and tissues are not regenerated. Under these circumstances, we tend to age more quickly and feel less fit than we should. We are not exactly sick, but neither are we in vibrant health.

Raw foods are a rich source of enzymes. Without enzymes, food could not be digested. It is the enzymes in foods and those manufactured by our own bodies that help convert foods into new cells and tissues. We need the enzymes found in fresh, raw foods; with these, the energy potential of our cells is boosted and we spare the body the extra work to avoid depleting its own reserves. Overcooking quite simply destroys living enzymes.

Raw foods have unique cleansing properties. They reduce the burden of wastes that the body has to deal with and eliminate those already stored in the tissues. With their high potassium content, raw foods gradually detoxify the body and play a major role in eliminating the congestive buildup of cellulite. Raw foods also supply the valuable fiber so important for sweeping the whole digestive system free of wastes.

Besides their vitamin, mineral, and high water content, raw foods contain valuable antioxidants that heal and repair tissues (more about this later).

Does this mean we should eat only raw foods? No. But every effort should be made to eat fresh, raw foods as often as possible. A diet is not balanced unless generous portions of raw foods are included. This can be accomplished quite easily by eating fresh, raw fruits throughout the day and by emphasizing fresh vegetable salads as delicious accompaniments to meals. And always try to start a meal with something raw: crudités, salad, fresh fruit, or fresh fruit salad. Freshly extracted juices and blenderized fruit are also wonderfully easy and delicious ways to use raw foods. At least 30 percent of the food we eat should be raw—more would be even better.

FRESH FRUIT AND RAW VEGETABLE JUICES

By juicing fresh fruits and raw vegetables with a juice extractor, we derive maximum benefits from them. Juices are replete with vitamins, minerals, and vital enzymes. Freshly extracted juices are digested in a matter of minutes and assimilated into the system in only a few more. And they taste wonderful!

Fresh juices are excellent thirst quenchers, cleansers, and tonics that have a remarkably revitalizing effect upon the entire body. Their purifying and detoxifying properties are unsurpassed: They purify the blood, neutralize the wastes cast off by our cells, and help build new, healthy tissues.

A juice extractor should be part of your kitchen equipment just as your blender is. The taste of fresh juices has nothing in common with commercial juices, nor is there any comparison in nutritive value. If you have never sampled the freshly extracted juices of fruits and vegetables, you're in for a real treat. Try to include a large glass or two in your diet every day. This is a superb way to load up on valuable potassium—and give your body an internal bath of health and vitality.

When juicing, fruits and vegetables should not be mixed. There are, however, two exceptions to this rule: Apples can be mixed with vegetables and celery mixes with fruit. When adding greens—spinach, kale, broccoli, green pepper, Romaine lettuce, and so forth—use one-quarter greens, the rest carrots and a little apple juice if desired. Apples can always be used to improve the flavor of otherwise bitter or strong-tasting juices.

Although carrot juice is quite popular, it's even more beneficial when combined with other vegetables. You might try carrot-celery-cucumber, carrot-broccoli-apple, or carrot-tomato-celery. These are only suggestions; the combinations are virtually limitless, so be creative.

Here are some tips to help you enjoy the maximum benefits freshly extracted juices have to offer:

- Do not peel. Exception is made, of course, for those fruits with coarse skins, such as pineapple, citrus, and the like. Simply scrub with a vegetable brush under cold running water.
- Cut up fruits and vegetables just prior to juicing.
- Juice fruits that are firm. Eat them when they're soft and ripe.
- Drink juices immediately after extraction. Otherwise, they oxidize and lose their vitamin content along with their highly perishable enzymes.

- Juices are best drunk fresh. If necessary, however, they may be kept in an airtight container in the refrigerator for a few hours.
- Be sure to drink them in small sips. Do not gulp down.
- For better assimilation, always drink fresh juices on an empty stomach—never with or following a meal.
- As much as possible, try to keep your juicer handy, always ready to be used. If it's too much of a hassle to pull it out of the cabinet, you're likely not to use it as often.

To learn more about the wonderful properties and possibilities of fresh juices, check with your local health food store. There are many excellent books on juicing.

BLENDERIZED FRUIT

A delicious—and easy—way to eat fruit is to blenderize it. There are some big advantages in eating fruit this way: more of the nutrients are assimilated, all the fiber is retained, and you derive maximum nutritional benefits. The blender does the "chewing" for you. You can also eat a variety of fruits at once.

Mix two or three kinds of fruits to enhance the taste of the purée. This will also allow you to utilize fruits that are either not very tasty or not sweet enough on their own. You can also vary the consistency of the mixture—certain fruits are naturally more "creamy" while others are more "liquidy." Peaches and apples, for example, have a smooth texture while grapes yield juicy liquid. You may also want to add a bit of plain yogurt, a couple of teaspoons per serving, for a creamier texture.

A blenderized "purée" makes an excellent appetizer. You can serve it in an elegant cup or bowl decorated with a few raspberries or some slices of kiwi or strawberry. You may want to top it with chopped nuts or grated coconut.

Here are a few delicious combinations to try:

- One small apple, one peach or nectarine, and a handful of strawberries or raspberries.
- A slice of fresh pineapple, half a mango or papaya, and a kiwi.

Use the intermittent cycle of the blender to keep too much air from getting mixed in. If necessary, add a tablespoon or so of fresh juice to make the blending easier. Or begin with the juicier fruits—berries or grapes, for example—blend, and then add the other fruits.

"Smoothies" are thick drinks made in a blender. To make them more liquidy, you can omit the banana or use only half. Be sure all fruits are ripe.

Fruit Smoothie

> 1 cup fresh juice
> 1 fresh or frozen banana
> 1 or 2 cups fresh fruit of your choice

Combine all ingredients and blend.

SALADS

Salads mean more than lettuce. It is true, however, that a simple salad made with crisp greens can be absolutely delicious either at the start of a meal or after the main course, but eating a salad before the main course has its advantages. It serves to fill you up and thus keeps you from overeating. Also, it stimulates your digestive juices, especially if you use a squeeze of fresh lemon. By appeasing your appetite with a salad, you can eat more slowly instead of devouring the main course.

Salads give you the perfect opportunity to eat a large variety of raw vegetables. The choice is quite broad—in addition to the usual lettuce, radishes, and tomatoes, you will want to try zucchini, broccoli, cauliflower, onions, scallions, green and red peppers, mushrooms, avocado, fresh peas, cucumbers, celery, and sprouts. Crunchy cooked vegetables make a delicious addition also: try beets, string beans, and asparagus. Always try to have at least four or five vegetables in your salad.

There are some delicious finishing touches that can give your salads extra flavor as well as extra nutrients—for example, grated apple, grated carrot, currants, seeds, nuts, rice, bulgur, couscous, and buckwheat. Legumes such as beans, chick-peas, and lentils and grains such as rice, bulgur, and couscous can also serve as the "base" for a salad—the raw or cooked vegetables are then added. Such a dish makes a complete, nutrition-packed meal by itself.

Here are some other suggestions for salads:

■ Potatoes make delicious salads, but not the conventional potato salad available in restaurants, salad bars, and delicatessens. This kind is to be avoided completely. Instead, try cooking red potatoes or new potatoes, cut in pieces, and serve with a lean dressing. This is a refreshing salad for summer meals.

- Cold meats that you cook at home make a good addition to a salad—especially chicken, turkey, and perhaps very lean roast beef occasionally. Stay away from ham, however, as it is too salty and too fat. The same is true for "bacon bits."
- Hard-boiled egg whites can make a delicious addition to a salad and lend some extra flavor and texture. Cheese, too, if you use it very sparingly—Swiss cheese is preferable to cheddar, which is very salty. A sprinkle of freshly grated Parmesan cheese will really spice up a salad.
- As for the greens themselves, remember that there's a wide choice out there. Try not to rely on the usual iceberg lettuce as it does not offer much in the way of nutrition. Instead, try Boston lettuce, Romaine, fresh spinach, chicory, watercress, cabbage, endive, and arugula.

Salad Dressings

Dressings should be dribbled, not poured, over salads. Their purpose is to enhance flavor and bring out the taste of the salad. We all tend to use too much dressing at times, and often this destroys what could otherwise be a lean, wholesome meal.

Most commercial dressings are not recommended. They contain far too much fat, salt, and sugar—as well as many chemical additives. While the reduced-calorie and "no-oil" dressings seem like a good idea, they contain even more salt than the regular ones as well as more chemicals—so much so that they actually "taste" and "smell" chemical. They are not a good alternative since in solving one problem they lead to others. You're merely trading offenders here.

Some suggestions for making your own salad dressings include:

- Whenever possible, try to use fresh lemon juice instead of vinegar. It's much better for you as it contains vitamin C and aids digestion.
- Add yogurt to a basic vinaigrette to make a creamy dressing. Or, use yogurt as a base to which you can add lemon juice and Dijon mustard.

Salad Bars

These can be a godsend or a disaster—depending on how you handle them. Usually, there are far too many choices, many of them laden with mayonnaise, salt, sugar, and fats. Be very selective here.

- First of all, avoid all the "prepared" choices, such as potato salad, macaroni salad, and the like.
- Select from the wide range of fresh vegetables, such as lettuce, green pepper, tomatoes, carrots, onions, broccoli, and cauliflower. Try to include some red kidney beans or some chick-peas if available.
- A few croutons are okay, but skip the bacon bits.
- Watch out for the dressings! These can ruin your meal. Stick to fresh lemon juice or oil and vinegar. Or better yet, take your own dressing from home.
- If it's available, help yourself to a slice or two of whole-grain bread. This will complete a wholesome main course.

SOUPS

Soup can be very good food—the soup you make yourself that is. Canned and dry soups are so high in sodium that one cup supplies the requirements for an entire day, and they contain many chemicals that you have no use for. As a matter of fact, some contain no natural ingredients at all; they are entirely chemical.

Homemade soups, on the other hand, are terrific. They can be a rich source of minerals, potassium in particular, since the cooking water is not discarded, and a high source of fiber as well. And homemade soups are very satisfying.

If you eat soup at the beginning of a meal, you will be less likely to overeat. As a main course, soup is also excellent, especially if accompanied by a slice of whole-grain bread or a muffin and a green salad. In fact, this combination constitutes an ideal meal.

When preparing soups, use a variety of fresh vegetables to which you may add beans, peas, lentils, brown rice, barley, or pasta. The list of ingredients, of course, is endless, so try to vary your recipes to avoid monotony.

The ways to serve soup are also extensive. Hot soups are comforting in winter, and chilled soups are refreshing in summer. You can prepare a creamy soup in your blender. A thick, hearty soup can be served as a stew.

Raw Soups

These soups—made from delicious, fresh, raw ingredients—comprise a category all their own. Because the vegetables are not cooked or tampered with in any way, they retain all their vitamins, minerals, and essential enzymes just as if you were eating them raw. Fiber content is also intact, so you reap its benefits as well.

The following are merely suggestions for raw soups. Just as with fresh juices, the options are unlimited, and you should experiment freely. For a chunkier kind of soup, set the blender on a slow speed; a medium setting may be used for a creamier texture. Fresh vegetable juice or filtered water may serve as a base. Avocado may be added to any raw soup for a really creamy consistency—and should be added last.

Fresh Asparagus Soup

1 lb. fresh asparagus
1 stalk celery
1 tbsp. parsley
Pinch of oregano and thyme
1 tbsp. almonds
1 tbsp. olive oil
1 tbsp. kelp

Combine all the ingredients and blend.

Creamy Broccoli Soup

1 cup fresh broccoli
1 clove garlic
1 cup alfalfa sprouts
1 tbsp. olive oil
½ tsp. kelp
1 cup filtered water
½ avocado

Blend all ingredients except avocado. Add avocado and blend again.

Cucumber Purée

- 1 cucumber
- 1 small zucchini
- 1 avocado
- 1 cup filtered water
- Fresh lemon or lime juice
- 1 clove garlic

Combine all ingredients and blend.

All of the above soups, and any that you invent on your own, may be served as is, at room temperature, or chilled. In cool weather, however, you may wish to heat the soup a bit. A warm version may be made by simply using warm filtered water in the blending process or by placing the soup in the top of a double boiler and heat only as much as necessary. Avoid direct contact with the heat source so as not to destroy the delicate enzymes.

DRIED FRUIT

Dried fruit is high in both potassium and fiber and, when eaten in moderation, is very beneficial to a healthy digestive tract. However, they *are* high in calories, albeit healthy, nutritious calories.

Dried fruits make a perfect addition to many foods, such as homemade cookies, pancake batter, breakfast cereals, homemade breads and muffins, and even salads. They are an ideal sweetener because they are highly concentrated; you don't need very much.

Excellent for snacking, most dried fruits provide quick energy and "brain fuel." You would be much better off eating a few pieces of dried fruit instead of a doughnut, a pastry, or a candy bar during a mid-morning break or late-afternoon slump. A handful of raisins or currants—or a few prunes, figs, dates, or apricots—will do the trick.

Pineapple and papaya are two fruits you must be careful with. Both are beneficial in their natural state but loaded with added sugar when dried. These are practically in the category of candy. It's possible to find pineapple and papaya dried without sugar, but it's difficult. Be cautious.

WHOLE GRAINS AND LEGUMES

These are the ideal foods around which to center your meal planning, and they should account for most of your daily calories. They are the very best energy sources because they are digested slowly and steadily. They also supply large amounts of fiber, bulk, and essential nutrients, which provide long-lasting satiety.

The whole grains—wheat, rice, oats, barley, millet, quinoa, and buckwheat—and the products made from them (breads, cereals, pasta) provide perfect "fuel" for the human body's metabolism. The same is true for legumes—dried beans, peas, and lentils—which are richer in protein than any other plant food. I should mention at this point that potatoes, though vegetables, fit into the category of "starch" because of their molecular structure.

Although starches were once thought of as fattening, we now know that this is simply not true. By themselves they are very low in fat calories (the bad guys). What makes them fattening is the way in which they are usually prepared and served: potatoes are fried or drowned in mayonnaise; beans are cooked with pork; pasta is accompanied by rich sauces laden with oil, salt, sugar, and fatty meats (not to mention the sauces made from heavy cream and butter).

When prepared properly, starches are easily digested and very satisfying. They provide high-quality nutrients, including protein, in just the right amounts and proportions. They are also easy to prepare and quite versatile.

For optimal nutrition, always accompany starches—rice, beans, pasta, potatoes—with a generous serving of fresh vegetables and a salad. Such a meal will provide you with all the necessary nutrients—protein (amino acids), essential fat, fiber, vitamins, minerals—you need to function and look your best.

Here are a few suggestions:

- A bed of brown rice makes an ideal base for steamed or stir-fried vegetables. Your local health food store probably carries many kinds of brown rice, including Basmati, an aromatic variety with a subtle nutlike flavor.
- Quinoa makes a light, delicious alternative to brown rice and cooks very quickly. To enhance the flavor, you may want to cook it in a vegetable broth.
- Couscous (a wheat product) has become quite popular during the past few years and can be served just like rice. There is a whole wheat variety available at health food stores.
- Barley, which is very high in fiber, can be added to almost any soup.
- Buckwheat groats or kasha also make an excellent base for steamed or stir-fried vegetables. Look for the whole-groat type.

- As for pasta, try to obtain the whole-grain varieties: buckwheat, corn, artichoke, whole wheat, quinoa, sesame—all available at health food stores.
- There is more to whole-grain bread than whole wheat. Try some of the interesting varieties that combine five, six, or seven different grains. Also look for sprouted-grain breads in health food stores. The ones that list the grains as the first ingredients are the ones you want—not the commercial products that are made primarily from flour.
- A plain baked potato served with a bit of whipped butter or yogurt, some vegetables, and a large green salad makes a delicious meal. For a change of pace, try sweet potatoes or yams served this way.
- Legumes are extremely versatile. While they make excellent soups (and this is how most people prepare them), you can do a lot more with them. They're great in salads. Hummus is a good example of using a legume, in this case chick-peas, as a base for dips. Also, legumes can be mashed and used as a tasty sandwich spread, and they can be sprouted. Be sure to use them regularly. (Most people think legumes require overnight soaking. This is not so. Here is a tip for easy cooking: Bring the dried beans to a boil for one minute, let stand one to three hours. Prepared this way, most beans will cook in a very short time.)

SPROUTS

Sprouts are a highly nutritious, easily digested, and inexpensive food, and many grains, beans, and seeds can be sprouted. Adzuki, alfalfa, barley, chick-peas, lentil, mung beans, millet, soybeans, sunflower, and wheat berries are among the most popular. Sprouting transforms these seeds, grains, and beans into high-energy foods packed with vital nutrients. When a seed is sprouted, its vitamin content is increased many times.

During the sprouting process, natural chemical changes occur. Starch begins to be broken down into simple sugars, fats to fatty acids, and protein into amino acids. Because of these changes, sprouts are already partially digested and therefore very easily assimilated.

Sprouts make an excellent addition to salads and sandwiches. When you add them to soup, casseroles, or any cooked meal, do so near the end as they require very little cooking, a few minutes at most.

Sprouts are widely available in supermarkets, greengrocers, and health food stores. Be sure to select the freshest and the crispiest—wilted sprouts lose their nutritional value—or grow your own. (The best and simplest way to do this is to use a "sprouter"—you can find various models in health food stores. This way, your sprouts will cost pennies and you will be assured they are fresh.) You can store them in the refrigerator in plastic bags or containers (always keep them covered); they will keep up to seven days.

NUTS AND SEEDS

This is an extremely valuable food group. Even though nuts and seeds are very high in calories, they are also high in the unsaturated fatty acids needed for healthy cells, and they are also a rich source of essential potassium and fiber. Used judiciously, they are an important food to include in your eating plan.

Nuts and seeds should be eaten fresh, raw, and unsalted. Roasting reduces their digestibility, while salting throws off the delicate sodium-potassium balance. Rancidity destroys their usefulness and even renders them harmful as the rancid fat generates free radicals.

Always buy nuts and seeds in small amounts that can be used quickly, and keep them refrigerated. Eat them while they're very fresh. It's a good idea to mix them in order to get a good balance of amino acids. They make excellent high-energy snacks and a delicious, crunchy addition to salads.

WHAT ABOUT FIBER?

Fiber is plant material that cannot be digested by man. It is found in all unrefined grains, dried beans, and peas as well as in all fruits and vegetables. Because it is indigestible, it acts as a "broom" to sweep the entire digestive system of wastes and dead cells. It also slows down the digestion of complex carbohydrates, enabling their glucose to be released at a slower pace to maintain even levels of blood sugar. It prevents the "slumps"—those all too familiar feelings of hunger, irritability, and fatigue—resulting in more sustained energy and a better mood.

There are many different types of fiber—cellulose, hemicellulose, lignin, pectin, and gums—each with its own ability to keep you well. All are important. Fiber is the antidote to the most common problem resulting from our modern diet of refined, processed foods, namely constipation. It aids elimination by adding bulk to waste material through water absorption. By promoting "rapid transit" through the digestive tract, fiber reduces the chances for bacteria and other unhealthy situations to develop.

There seems to be some rather common but mistaken notions regarding fiber. Many people tend to regard fiber as an item limited to breakfast foods—muffins, granola, commercial cereals, and the like. This simply is not the case. Fiber, like protein, is everywhere, and the best strategy is to eat a variety of high-fiber foods throughout the day. That way, you'll hit on all the different types of fiber and reap all the benefits that these foods have to offer. Sprinkling a little bran or wheat germ on food in the morning and then ignoring your fiber needs for the rest of the day simply does not work. Keep in mind, too, that animal products, including meat, poultry, dairy items, eggs, fish, and shellfish, contain no fiber at all.

All unprocessed plant foods are extremely high in dietary fiber. If you follow the recommendations in the anti-cellulite way of eating, you are certain to get plenty of valuable, natural fiber from the very best sources. In other words, "eating right" will satisfy the need for this important substance without unnecessary calculations or worry.

WATER... A MUCH NEGLECTED NUTRIENT

Next to oxygen, water is our most vital nutrient. Unfortunately, it is also our most neglected one. While we could survive for quite a while without food, we would last only a few days without water. Water regulates body temperature, brings oxygen and nutrients to cells, carries away waste products, lubricates joints, and keeps the immune system working. In addition to performing all of these vital functions, water is the best moisturizer of all: It hydrates the system from within, keeping tissues and skin supple, moist, and youthful.

Drinking plenty of water is absolutely essential in fighting cellulite. It is the ultimate cleanser of the body, the only healthy diuretic. Water flushes out the system through perspiration and urination, and thus cleans the cells of wastes that impede microcirculation. Without sufficient water, the tissue sludge that causes cellulite is allowed to accumulate in the spaces between cells. And this is exactly what we wish to avoid or clear up. Water in proper quantities and at the right times will aid tremendously in this process of cleansing the internal environment. Think of water as an internal bath or shower.

Water accounts for approximately two-thirds of the body or about 65 percent of its weight. This water is distributed in a relatively constant fashion among the body's three fluid compartments: inside the cells, outside the cells in the interstitial spaces, and in the blood vessels. Every single cell of the body depends upon water to carry out its functions. Water is essential to the digestion and absorption of food from the gastrointestinal tract as well as the elimination of digestive wastes.

Not only does water accelerate the elimination of cellulite, but it is essential to weight management as well. For those who have a tendency to retain fluid, water helps flush it out. There is a common but mistaken belief that water retention and high water consumption are related. This is not true. It is sodium, or salt, that encourages this condition by attracting fluids to tissues; drinking pure water counteracts this tendency.

How much water do we really need? There are those who advocate drinking water by the gallon; I don't agree with this. Keep in mind our key principle of "moderation" here as in all matters: The harmonies of the body are best served with sensible amounts of food and water. Six to eight glasses of water a day are mandatory. You might need more if you are exercising vigorously, perspire a great deal, or are under severe stress, but six to eight glasses is the minimum and they should be spread throughout the day.

The best way to drink water is in small amounts. Gulping should always be avoided. When water is allowed to trickle slowly through the system, it performs its many functions with greater efficiency. Half a glass every hour or one glass every two hours or so, taken in small sips, is ideal. In this way, water best nourishes, purifies, detoxifies, and hydrates. Swallowing large amounts at a time produces a temporary overload, which puts a strain on the kidneys and passes right through the system without doing its job properly.

Remember, too, that foods naturally high in water content—fruits and vegetables contain on average 80–90 percent water—form the basis of our anti-cellulite diet. Thus, by eating plenty of foods high in water content and by drinking water throughout the day, we are assured of meeting our body's needs.

It is better not to drink with meals as this tends to dilute digestive juices. And "washing down" your foods with liquids actually lets you eat more while preventing you from chewing properly. Drinking water with a meal is permissible if you take very small sips. But remember, *very small sips* at a time—no gulping.

Here are some additional tips for drinking more water:

- Always drink a large glass of water first thing in the morning, before anything else.

- Keep water nearby when working, reading, or relaxing. It also helps to use an attractive glass or goblet that will entice you to sip frequently.
- Make it a habit to drink water liberally before, during, and after exercise. This is essential to replace the water lost through perspiration.
- When you pass a water fountain, always help yourself to a long, quenching drink.
- Perk up your water from time to time with a squeeze of fresh lemon.
- Finally, substitute water for other beverages when possible. You will find very soon that you are drinking more water and fewer diet sodas, cups of coffee, and nonherbal teas, which actually "leech" needed water from your system by acting as diuretics.

A Word About the Quality of Your Water

Thousands of chemicals find their way into our water. Some, such as chlorine, are added for our protection, to destroy bacteria and other harmful substances. Others form in the chlorination process as the synthetic by-products of chlorine. While the quality of tap water varies greatly throughout the country and the world, nearly all water supplies today are tainted by chemicals to some degree, even well water in rural areas. Many of these chemicals enter the water supply through unavoidable ground seepage as a result of the substances used in heavy industry, agriculture, and waste disposal.

It is to our advantage to safeguard the water we drink as well as the water we use in cooking (as boiling water may actually concentrate contaminants). One simple way to remove the vast majority of chemicals and other undesirable elements is by using a water filter that attaches to your faucet. Such a unit in your own kitchen is practically indispensable and a wise investment in your long-term health. Be sure to change the cartridge often; as a general rule, twice as often as manufacturers suggest.

What About Bottled Mineral Water?

Long-time European favorites, these are becoming increasingly popular in the states as well, and are especially practical for your drinking needs when outside the home. Many come in attractive bottles that can be easily carried around. As for naturally effervescent ones, try to keep those for special occasions, as it is not a good idea to drink carbonated liquids in large amounts. They do, however, make a nice refreshing treat with a twist of lemon or lime and a perfect substitute to an alcoholic beverage. They are best sipped slowly.

MEAL PLANNING IDEAS

The anti-cellulite way to eat is actually quite simple. Remember, this is not a diet; it's a permanent way to eat. You need not limit the ingredients nor the amounts—within reasonable limits, of course. If you stick with the right foods and apply the proper eating principles outlined at the end of this chapter, you can't go wrong. You'll feel neither hungry nor deprived. These meals are satisfying, tasty, completely nutritious, and very enjoyable. And once you get used to eating this way, it will become second nature.

About Breakfast

The food you eat in the morning is the fuel your body uses until lunch. Breakfast does not necessarily have to be large, but it must contain the right nutrients. A good way to start is to drink a glass of freshly extracted fruit juice such as orange, grapefruit, or pineapple—or to eat fresh fruit: some luscious slices of mango or papaya, fresh juicy berries, a handful of grapes, or some kiwi slices.

The choices now are wide open in terms of what you may want to have for the meal itself. Cereals are considered the new breakfast "staple," and a well-chosen, well-prepared cereal makes an excellent breakfast item. Commercial cereals such as shredded wheat, puffed rice, puffed wheat, or grape nuts are fine. A health food store will offer many more varieties. All can be mixed with low-fat or skim milk or plain yogurt and raisins or currants or dates for sweetener. Another alternative that will give you tasty variety: to 4 ounces of plain yogurt, add some cut up figs or prunes, some seeds—sunflower, sesame—and a few chopped walnuts or almonds, and a spoonful or two of cereal.

Whole-grain toast with low-fat cheese or a little whipped butter and "fruit only" jam can be accompanied with a glass of low-fat or skim milk (especially if you skip the cheese). Occasionally, you can also prepare oven-baked French toast from whole-grain bread or some delicious buckwheat pancakes (buckwheat happens to be excellent for circulation).

No one says that you must eat breakfast as soon as you get out of bed. You can delay a few hours if you like. Many people are not hungry first thing in the morning, and there are many reasons for this—a late dinner the night before and/or a dinner that was too heavy. At night, our bodily processes, including digestion, slow down considerably, so we may still be digesting a meal from the night before when we wake up. This is one more reason to try to eat dinner no later than seven in the evening.

Here are two more breakfast suggestions that are simple and may really fit the bill if you're not too hungry or if a real "sit down" breakfast is not your style.

High-Energy Shake

½   cup low-fat or skim milk
½   cup juice or fresh juicy fruit
2–4 tbsp. plain yogurt
½   banana (preferably frozen)
A handful of berries

Combine all ingredients and blend.

For a dairy-free version, replace the milk and yogurt with soy milk (available at health food stores) or almond milk (made with water and a few almonds).

For those people on the go, the ultimate "portable" breakfast is a handful of almonds and a few dates with a small glass of milk or some plain yogurt—a perfectly adequate breakfast.

If you're hungry in the middle of the morning, have a large glass of freshly extracted fruit or vegetable juice or a piece of fruit.

Lunch

Now is the time to emphasize vegetables in the form of large, crisp salads, delicious sandwiches, and nourishing soups. Of course, as far as salads go, a generous selection of fresh fruit is perfectly all right, too, but at lunchtime, it's a good idea to accompany this mix with some low-fat cottage cheese or yogurt to supply added protein and to make your salad more sustaining.

A big, fresh salad makes the perfect lunch, especially with a slice or two of whole-grain bread. You can toss a seasonal mix of vegetables—not just the usual lettuce and tomato. As we've seen in the salad section, the possibilities are limitless.

Sandwiches are the traditional lunch fare, and you can put together some great ones on your own—or find appealing, nutritious varieties on many menus. Whole-grain bread or whole-wheat pita can first be spread with mashed beans or hummus, then filled with crisp raw vegetables and a generous bouquet of sprouts. A popular version of this is the "California" sandwich: sliced avocado or guacamole, tomatoes, cucumber, and sprouts—with a smear of mayonnaise.

Another delicious meal for colder weather is a bowl of hearty soup, a small salad, and a slice or two of whole-grain bread.

And if by mid-afternoon you're hungry and want a snack, try a large glass of freshly extracted fruit or vegetable juice or a piece of fruit.

Dinner

Lunch and dinner are really interchangeable, but here are some additional suggestions. When at home, soups and salads can be whipped up easily—and you can make clever use of leftovers to add variety. For example, a dinner of brown rice and steamed or stir-fried vegetables is perfect, and the next evening you can use the leftover rice in your salad. The same is true of lean chicken, which you might have one evening with steamed or stir-fried vegetables and the next evening as a delicious garnish for your salad.

Other options for dining at home or in a restaurant include:

- Pasta with a light sauce and a generous helping of crisply cooked vegetables and a salad.
- Broiled or poached fish with fresh cooked vegetables and/or a large salad.
- An omelette with a salad (this is also a great option for lunch, especially when eating in a restaurant with limited selections).
- A baked potato with a generous serving of steamed or stir-fried vegetables and a small salad is a favorite with many people.
- Vegetable-based meals, garnished with small amounts of chicken or turkey if you like, prepared in a wok also make an excellent choice.

This list of suggestions is obviously only a partial one. Remember, you are *not* on a diet. Make large use of the many excellent cookbooks available now with recipes for wholesome meals made from fresh, lean, nutrient-rich foods that are easy to prepare and low in salt, fat, and sugar.

If you desire a snack at bedtime, your best choice is an apple.

Special Restorative Foods

TISSUE REPAIR

Firm, smooth skin depends upon a healthy supply of collagen. Made up of protein and the major structural molecule of the body, collagen is what gives the skin its elasticity, resiliency, and contour. As stated in Chapter 1, collagen begins to break down when we're in our early twenties. It is not merely the passage of time, however, that brings about this deterioration. Most of the damage results from errors in lifestyle. Not only can we prevent future damage, but we can gradually undo some of the existing damage with certain nutrients.

FREE RADICALS AND TISSUE DAMAGE

Free radicals, or oxidation radicals, play a major role in tissue breakdown. The process known as "cross-linking," the fusion of protein molecules under certain circumstances, is largely responsible for the characteristically uneven appearance of skin on thighs and buttocks. These areas of the body can appear prematurely old and devitalized due to cross-linked tissue, which results in sagging or draping of surface skin very often accompanied by deep pits and hollows.

It is true that free radicals are generated constantly as a natural function of body chemistry, and we do need a certain amount of controlled oxidation. But an excess of free radicals can lead to the kind of tissue damage described here.

Some sources of damaging free radicals are:

- High-fat foods
- Overeating—the more food you metabolize, the more free radicals you generate
- Rapid weight loss
- Environmental pollution
- Internal pollution caused by cigarette smoking, excessive consumption of alcohol and caffeine, drugs, stress, constipation, and illness

The Healing Foods

Fortunately, Nature has provided a powerful antidote to free radicals in the form of antioxidants. These substances deactivate the potentially dangerous free radicals before they can damage vital cells. The body manufactures its own antioxidants in the enzymes superoxide dismutase (SOD) and glutathione peroxidase.

There are also many natural antioxidants in food that can come to our rescue. Among the most effective are beta-carotene (vitamin A), vitamin C, vitamin E, and the mineral selenium. Also, to manufacture its own antioxidants, the body needs adequate supplies of zinc, copper, and manganese.

Antioxidants are the natural healers of tissue and can help repair damage to our cells as we age. In fact, a great deal of what we call "premature aging" can be prevented or arrested with the aid of these effective healing substances. We can protect ourselves from free radical damage by making certain that we get abundant natural antioxidants from food sources. Some excellent foods to include in your diet are:

Beta-carotene
Sweet potatoes, carrots, spinach, broccoli, leafy green vegetables, yellow vegetables, red pepper, cantaloupe, papaya, and apricots.

Vitamin C
Citrus fruits, cantaloupe, tomatoes, potatoes, broccoli, Brussels sprouts, cabbage, cauliflower, kale, and sweet peppers.

Vitamin E
Whole grains, leafy green vegetables, wheat germ, wheat germ oil, sunflower seeds, almonds, pecans, and cold-pressed vegetable oils.

Selenium
Whole-grain cereals and breads, wheat germ, asparagus, broccoli, onions, garlic, tomatoes, cabbage, egg yolks, seafood, and milk.

Zinc, Copper, Manganese
Whole grains, seeds, nuts, and legumes.

AN EXTRA TIP TO ENHANCE COLLAGEN RENEWAL
Under normal circumstances, about half our collagen supply is replaced every five to seven years. We can actually step up this process—and also undo some cross-linking—by including a few special fruits in our diet. Pineapple and papaya in particular contain the valuable collagen renewing enzymes bromelain and papain. Mango and kiwi also contain compa-

rable enzymes that contribute to the formation of new, healthy collagen fibers. All four of these tasty fruits should be eaten raw and at their peak of seasonal ripeness.

You may eat these fruits in their natural state or blend them in a purée, which makes a refreshing breakfast item or a delicious snack.

A word of caution: Try not to overindulge to the point of causing soreness in the mouth. Also, if you have an ulcer, these fruits will slow down its healing and should be avoided.

STRENGTHEN YOUR CAPILLARIES

Research in Europe has shown that women with cellulite often have weak capillaries. As explained earlier, it is the excess seepage from weakened capillaries that initially encourages the cellulite-forming process. Thus, strengthening the walls of the capillaries will improve overall microcirculation and reduce this tendency.

Certain nutrients, namely the "bioflavonoids" and vitamin C, are particularly helpful in improving capillary function. Not entirely by coincidence, many of the foods that help in building stronger capillaries also contain high concentrations of potassium.

Bioflavonoids are natural substances that occur in fruits and vegetables, particularly those with vitamin C. These two elements work together to strengthen capillaries and make them more resilient. Because of their regulating effect on permeability of the capillaries, bioflavonoids were originally identified as vitamin P. This nutritional element along with vitamin C keeps collagen, the structural material of capillaries, in good shape. It also enhances the action of vitamin C and prevents it from oxidizing.

The best sources of bioflavonoids are the citrus fruits—oranges, grapefruits, lemons, limes—eaten with as much of the pith or white pulp as possible, and grapes, apricots, strawberries, papaya, black currants, plums, cantaloupe, and cherries. Some vegetable sources are broccoli, red peppers, and tomatoes. All fruits and most vegetables, of course, should be eaten raw. Among whole grains, buckwheat or kasha is the best choice. And even one of our most popular "seasonings," paprika, contains vitamin P.

Special Situations . . .
and Some Tips

EATING OUT

Restaurant food is generally too high in the very things you want to avoid: salt, fat, and sugar. On top of that, many restaurants depend upon a certain number of processed foods to supplement the menu. However, with a little awareness and some skillful juggling, you can learn to make choices that will not wreak havoc upon your eating plan.

Dining out can and should be a pleasant experience. It is an integral part of the American lifestyle and a simple fact of life for many people. For social and business reasons, a significant number of Americans find themselves eating in restaurants several times a week. We can make the best of this experience by keeping a few things in mind and by learning to make prudent choices even with the most lackluster menus. Here are some suggestions that may help.

- Eat a piece of fresh fruit or some raw vegetables *before* you go to a restaurant to take the edge off your appetite.
- Avoid temptations by asking the waiter to "hold" what you don't want to eat. Many meals are accompanied by french fries, cole slaw, potato chips, pickles, and so on. If these things are not in front of you, you won't miss them. Ask for more nutritious substitutes, and if none are available, just stick with the main item.
- Plan ahead when possible. Try to decide in advance what you are going to eat so that you won't be tempted to make wrong choices when you scan the menu.
- Be very specific when you order. Don't be afraid to ask how certain foods are prepared—whether they are fried, baked, poached, or broiled. Request vegetables that are steamed, meat and poultry prepared without oil or butter, and fresh, not canned, fruit. Specify that you would like the gravy, sauce, or dressing on the side so that you can control the portions. Above all, don't be self-conscious about ordering this way: These requests are neither unusual nor difficult to fill, and more and more people are asking for them.
- Try to begin your meal with a simple green salad or fresh fruit. Either one of these will help take the edge off your appetite and

prevent you from attacking the bread basket. Moreover, this will satisfy the requisite for including raw food with your meal, thus providing necessary enzymes for proper digestion and easy assimilation.

- A salad and an appetizer or two can often suffice as a complete meal. This will also satisfy your need for variety.
- When eating bread, skip the butter or spread it very thin.
- Never order "creamed" anything.
- Choose restaurants carefully. Avoid those that have menus limited to high-calorie, fat-laden foods.
- Never order "fried" anything. Broiled, baked, roasted, poached, and steamed foods are the healthiest and best.
- Unless you are very disciplined and/or not famished, you should avoid the all-you-can-eat kind of establishment. The same goes for buffets, although these can be wonderful in the sense of allowing you to make your own nutritious selections.
- When eating in Chinese restaurants, ask them to hold the MSG (monosodium glutamate). Also, stay away from the noodles that are placed on the table (they're too greasy).

BROWN BAGGING

If you work outside the home, try to get into the habit of brown bagging. It can work wonders for your health, your figure, your energy level, and your budget. For one thing, your efficiency level will improve dramatically as the food you eat at lunch is reflected in your mood throughout the afternoon.

Also, you are assured of nutritious foods, fewer calories, less fat, sugar, and salt—and more vitamins, minerals . . . and choices.

A few suggestions for packing your own lunch include:

- For a salad, put all the dry ingredients in a plastic bag with the dressing in a separate container (or keep your dressing at work). Mix your salad just before you are ready to eat.
- Pita or "pocket" sandwiches are very portable. To prevent the bread from becoming soggy, add the stuffing at the last minute.
- Soups and stews can be transported in a wide-mouth thermos.
- Use leftovers from home creatively. You can invent interesting new combinations to suit your preferences and your needs.

SNACKS

Snacking is okay if you reach for the right foods. Here are some suggestions that will not interfere with your healthy eating plan.

- Fresh fruit
- Crudités
- Homemade shakes and smoothies
- Freshly extracted vegetable juice
- Plain low-fat yogurt (4 oz.) with a teaspoon of currants or fresh fruit
- Plain, air-popped popcorn
- Ready-to-eat dry cereals without any added sweetener or salt: spoon-size shredded wheat, puffed wheat, puffed rice, puffed corn, and oat cereals
- A rice cake with "fruit only" jam
- A small homemade muffin
- Whole-grain bread or toast with "fruit only" jam or one ounce of low-fat cheese
- Small amounts of dried fruit or trail mix
- Unsalted nuts and seeds
- Unsalted whole-wheat pretzels and other healthy variations of common snack items available at health food stores

DESSERTS

As a general rule: skip dessert.

On occasion, you may have sherbet or ice milk—for example, when eating out. These do not offer much in the way of nutrition, but they are certainly better than ice cream, rich pastries, cakes, and pies. Such desserts have no place in a healthy diet and give you nothing but loads of sugar and fat.

A small serving of plain low-fat yogurt with raisins or currants and maybe a few chopped nuts as a topping makes a refreshing, satisfying dessert now and then.

Home-baked cakes and cookies made with whole-grain flour and a minimum of sugar—or better yet, dried fruit for sweetener—are acceptable and can make a nice change from time to time. Health food stores and other reliable sources also provide such desserts.

As for commercial frozen yogurts and tofu ice cream, forget about them entirely. What began as a good idea has deteriorated into overly sweet products that are no better than the regular ones.

Fruit "Ice Cream"

These make an excellent substitute for those who cannot do without ice cream. They are also wonderfully refreshing in hot weather.

- Fruit sherbet: Mix peaches, berries (strawberries, raspberries, and/ or blueberries), pears, and seedless grapes with enough apple juice or water to blend. Then freeze. For a creamier variety, blend again, and freeze.
- For an instant version, simply put a combination of frozen fruit (that you freeze yourself, of course) in the blender and add just enough water to blend easily. Peaches, grapes, melons, bananas, and berries make good choices. Remember to peel bananas and melons before freezing.

COOKING METHODS

The way in which you prepare foods greatly affects their nutritional value as well as their caloric content.

The secret with cooking is a gentle touch. Steaming is best. Vitamins are lost with boiling, but undercooked vegetables retain many, in some cases most, of their original nutrients. Always bake, broil, poach, or steam foods whenever possible. Pressure cooking is excellent, too.

With the exception of stews and soups, when the liquid is consumed along with the rest, avoid using large amounts of water when cooking. This is especially true for vegetables since most of the valuable vitamins and minerals, potassium especially, will be discarded with the excess water. When water is needed, use a minimum amount so that it will be absorbed during cooking. If there is any left, use it right away or save it for future use in soups. You can also drink any excess water from vegetable cooking—it's quite delicious.

Avoid frying foods. This changes their chemistry and makes them literally indigestible. It also produces dangerous free radicals. Frying furthermore adds unnecessary fats and calories to otherwise wholesome foods. Fried foods clog circulation. An exception is made for "stir frying" as this method uses a minimum of fat.

LIST OF STAPLES TO HAVE ON HAND AT ALL TIMES

This is not meant as a complete list to fill your pantry for all your culinary needs. Rather, it is a list of foods that you should have handy, not only to save time but to prevent you from making mistakes. It also allows you to prepare something nutritious at the last minute instead of reaching for the wrong foods.

- Vegetables: Carrots, onions, green and red peppers, avocados, and tomatoes plus a variety of fresh, leafy greens such as lettuce, endive, and watercress. (These keep well and make delicious salads as well as tasty sandwich items.)
- Potatoes: Idaho, red, and sweet
- Fruit: Always try to have a few of the "sturdy" types such as apples, certain varieties of pears, and bananas. Cantaloupes, too, are excellent and keep well. Of course, you should also have a wide range of fruits that are in season.
- Lemons: For salad dressings and steamed and stir-fried vegetables
- Grains: Buckwheat groats (kasha), rice (preferably brown), couscous, bulgur, quinoa, millet, and barley (nonpearled)
- Cereals: Both ready-to-eat and those that are prepared hot such as oatmeal and the like
- Pasta
- Dried beans and lentils
- Canned or frozen legumes: red kidney beans, chick-peas, lima beans, and so on
- Dried fruits: Raisins, prunes, currants, and apricots
- Unsalted nuts and seeds
- Unpopped popcorn
- Rice cakes
- Unsalted, whole-grain crackers
- Dairy products: Plain low-fat yogurt, cottage cheese (low-fat and unsalted if available), and low-fat or skim milk
- Canned fish: Water-packed tuna and salmon (When possible, try to get the no-salt varieties available in health food stores. If not, remember to rinse under water to de-salt.)

The "How to" of Eating Right

PROPER EATING PRINCIPLES

These are the principles that control "eating right." They are guidelines meant to ease or facilitate digestion and thereby allow better assimilation of essential nutrients.

- Fruits, vegetables, and whole grains should predominate in the ideal diet.
- The closer a food is to its natural state, the more nutritious it is.
- Keep your meals simple.
- Always try to eat something raw before eating something cooked. Also, use freshly squeezed lemon juice generously on cooked vegetables. It can also be added to many soups.
- Eat seasonally—for better taste and nutrition.
- Always accompany starches—rice, pasta, and potato dishes—with vegetables and/or a salad.
- When having meat or fish as the main course, serve with vegetables only. This makes for a much lighter meal than one served with rice or potatoes—and much easier to digest. It will be filling without producing a "stuffed" feeling. This is being done now in the better restaurants. A green salad with a lean dressing is the perfect accompaniment to such a meal.
- As for fruit, there are advantages to eating it ten to fifteen minutes before a meal (on an empty stomach). For one thing, it takes the edge off your appetite. Also, fruit digests very quickly, and it is assimilated much faster when eaten *before* a meal.
- As a rule, do not drink liquids with a meal. If you must have something to drink, make it a small glass and take tiny sips. *Never* gulp.
- If you are not hungry, or not entirely comfortable from the previous meal, postpone eating.
- Try to eat dinner no later than 7:00 P.M.—or three to four hours prior to bedtime.
- Avoid sweets after meals.
- If you give in occasionally to the temptation of fried food or fast food, be sure to include a great big salad along with it—use a generous squeeze of lemon and go easy on the dressing. This is especially sound advice for teenagers who often find themselves in fast-food establishments.

THE GOLDEN RULES OF NUTRITION

Eat Slowly and Chew Your Food Well

Almost everyone eats too fast—and this leads directly to eating too much. By eating slowly and by carefully chewing your food, you will actually eat less. The reason for this is simple: It takes about twenty minutes for your brain to signal your stomach that you're no longer hungry. It is the amount of food in your bloodstream, not in your stomach, that triggers the stop signal that means your body has had enough food to satisfy its needs.

Chewing properly is of utmost importance in the digestive process. There is no value to be derived from foods that are not digested as they only waste and spoil in the digestive tract adding toxins to an already overburdened system. The longer and better food is chewed, the more completely it is digested and assimilated. And what really matters is not only what you eat but what you absorb or assimilate. Thorough chewing releases digestive enzymes in the saliva that break down foods so that the stomach and intestines have less work to do.

Our mood also affects digestion. Rushed meals under tense conditions cannot possibly be digested properly. Emotions such as grief, fear, and anger also interfere with digestion. So, refrain from eating under the influence of tension and negative emotions. Always strive for a pleasant, relaxed atmosphere and a serene mood at mealtime.

Should you feel the need for a digestive aid, try eating an apple or some fresh pineapple. Papaya pills are also an effective aid to digestion and are available in health food stores and many drugstores. A cup of herbal tea such as mint chamomile works very well, too. Perhaps the best digestive aid of all is a brisk walk. Try it—you'll be amazed.

Eat Enough Food to Meet Your Body's Needs— Without Any Leftovers for Your Hips and Thighs

We actually need a lot less food than we think. Food is meant to bring essential nutrients to our trillions of cells. It is our fuel. Because your car needs gasoline to operate, would it occur to you to fill up the tank with more than it can hold? And more often than necessary? This may be a silly comparison, but it is exactly what most of us do every day, three times a day not counting snacks.

Eat sparingly! We should eat enough to meet our body's needs without having any left over for storage—or unwanted fat and cellulite. Food is not at all scarce in our society; if anything we have an excess. And it is this excess that is responsible for making us sick. There will always be plenty of food available in our lifetime, so why stuff ourselves?

As a society, we are overfed but often undernourished. We should eat foods that our bodies can use. Eating the right foods in the right amounts is really the name of the game. It's not that difficult.

Experiments on laboratory animals have shown that underfed animals have better resistance to disease and a longer lifespan than the overfed group. This is not to say that we should undereat or deprive ourselves of our nutritional needs. Rather, we should eat just the right amount.

The reason many of us eat too much is that we eat mostly, and in some cases exclusively, devitalized foods devoid of needed nutrients: vitamins, minerals, and enzymes. When deprived of the nutrients they need, our cells cry out for more food, so overeating is really a result of "undernourishing."

Overeating places a great deal of stress on the digestive system and takes a lot of energy. It also makes you feel sluggish for several hours afterward.

Once you begin to eat correctly, you will be surprised at how much less food you actually take in. After a proper meal, you will feel satisfied without the uncomfortable sensation of being stuffed. You will not be hungry again for several hours so you'll probably skip the usual snacks.

Seek Variety in Foods

This is your best assurance of getting all the necessary nutrients, including vitamins and minerals, that your body needs to function properly.

Try not to focus on any particular food. All categories are important. Your body needs a variety of foods, a balanced diet, to stay healthy. A diet that is out of balance is self-defeating; it will not make you permanently slender. If your cells lack essential nutrients, they will not have enough energy to burn fat. This is one of the reasons that diets usually fail. This is also why you feel tired and drained while dieting.

Variety also means avoiding boredom with certain foods. This can only lead to deficiencies and compensatory bingeing or overeating the wrong foods. Many of us tend to rely on the same old menus. Seek out new foods and new ways to prepare foods.

Select from all the categories—fruits, vegetables, whole grains, legumes—and vary your choices within each category. For example, your selection of fresh fruits should provide great variety each day. The same is true for vegetables. A good measure of variety here is color: If you have a wide assortment of colors on your plate, you have probably achieved effective variety. Colorful meals are generally nutritious meals. Food should be as aesthetically pleasing as it is nutritious.

Do Not Skip Meals

This is a very erroneous dieting notion—and a very common one. Many people skip meals in order to save on calories. This is a poor miscalculation.

Do not skip breakfast. If you reject food in the morning, your mood, energy level, and brain power will suffer throughout the day. Worse still, you'll be tempted by coffee-break time to indulge an appetite for all the wrong things, such as pastries, doughnuts, and candy bars. Breakfast skippers are lunch bingers—and spend the afternoon fighting somnolence and distention.

Do not skip lunch either. This is another silly trick to cut down on calories. When dinnertime comes, you'll be ready to devour anything in sight! And usually at high speed. What's more, if you skip lunch, by mid-afternoon, your blood sugar will be down—and so will you.

Eat on a regular timetable. Eating on an erratic schedule means you either eat when your body does not require food or you eat only when hunger pangs grow so strong that you consume far more food than you need. A regular schedule conditions your body to operate on the right amount of food at the right times. This does not necessarily mean the conventional three meals a day. In some cases, it is better to eat five or six small meals rather than one or two larger ones. The body will absorb a greater percentage of nutrients from a series of "mini-meals" than from a couple of more abundant ones. This is something you must determine for yourself by paying close attention to your body's needs and by organizing your meals around your daily routine.

Use Moderation at All Times

Moderation is a key word in this program. No extremes. You don't have to become a purist or a fanatic. You should not focus on one particular food category. Just because fruits and vegetables are good for you does not mean you should live on these alone. All food groups are important. And occasional "treats" and "cheats" are permissible as long as they do not become habits. In an otherwise healthy diet, these should be enjoyed without guilt.

When making changes in your diet, do it gradually. You will probably experience greater success if you have time to adapt to each change. And the changes are more likely to become permanent if you do not feel a sudden deprivation. While the "cold turkey" approach may work for some, it does not work for everyone. There is far less chance of relapse if you ease into a new lifestyle or new habits. If you go off your program from time to time, don't panic. Not all is lost. As soon as you can, get right back on track.

No one is expected to eat perfectly balanced meals every single day. Rather, think in terms of balancing food intake over a period of several days or a week. And remember, *it's what you eat on a regular basis that counts, not what you eat occasionally.*

Don't become a social bore or a party pooper. This makes other people uncomfortable—and you'll feel miserable, too. Have that sliver of delicious homemade pie or cake or fudge that someone has taken the time to prepare for you. Usually, just a taste of something that is yummy but not good for you will suffice.

And what do you do when you find yourself in a situation where there is absolutely nothing good for you to eat? Just make the best of it. You can nibble on a few things and then have something healthy when you get home. This will enable you to be gracious without courting disaster.

6

Effective Exercise

THE ROLE OF EXERCISE

Exercise shapes and maintains a lean, well-proportioned body. To get maximum results, two types of exercise are needed, as each has its own set of goals. *Body Shapers,* powerful isolation movements, zero in on specific parts of the body to sculpt and remodel as they firm, lift, and tighten. *Whole Body Conditioners,* often called "aerobics," speed metabolism, rev up circulation, and promote deep breathing. These two kinds of exercise work together to keep cellulite from settling in and spreading out.

Body Shapers... Your Muscles

Muscles give shape and contour to the body as well as tone and firmness. When muscles are exercised often and properly, as with these Body Shapers, they keep the arms firm and sinewy, the waistline tight and small, the abdomen flat, the thighs slim and shapely, and the buttocks round and uplifted. Unused muscle tissue tends to soften, weaken, and sag, creating unwanted bulges and a lumpy silhouette. If you are out of shape, or simply want to fine-tune your figure, the Body Shapers will give optimum results in minimum time.

Good muscle tone is also essential to efficient physiology. It is vital to

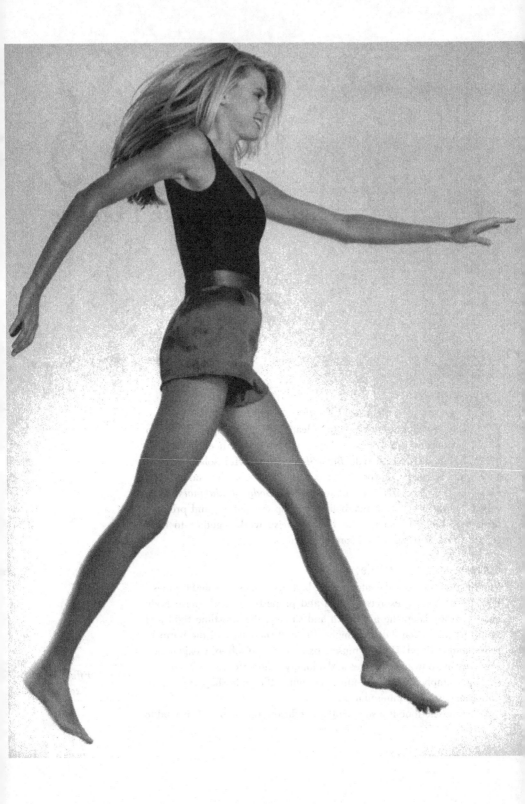

good circulation, which is responsible for transporting oxygen and nutrients to our trillions of cells and removing wastes from them. Muscles are also energy burners. The better shape they're in, the more efficient they will be at burning fat and calories. Muscles are toned only through systematic use. When not exercised regularly, they become flaccid and waste away. "Use it or lose it" definitely applies here. Undermuscled people are at a much higher risk of becoming "overfat"—and cellulite-prone.

As you are no doubt aware, your muscle-to-fat ratio is very important. The more muscle and the less fat you have, the higher your metabolism. This means that you will burn calories with greater speed and efficiency. It is not your overall weight that really matters, rather the proportion of fat to lean tissue. Greater muscle mass means more fat-burning enzymes in your body. Underused muscles lose these enzymes. Therefore, the way to improve your calorie-burning capacity is by improving your lean to fat ratio.

Generally speaking, women have more body fat than men. The amount of what is called "essential fat," that which is required for normal physiological functioning, is about 3 percent of total body weight for men and roughly 12 percent for women. Ideally, men should have 13–18 percent body fat, and women should have between 19 and 25 percent. Studies show that most men are between 22 and 24 percent— and the majority of women are between 26 and 34 percent.

Even if you are thin, you may be "overfat." Women who diet repeatedly are prime candidates for this. While they may "look" thin, if they have not exercised consistently they've lost a great deal of muscle tissue. The only way to increase muscle tissue while decreasing stored fat is by regular, systematic exercise along with careful eating. A metabolically efficient body is able to achieve and maintain a healthy muscle-to-fat ratio.

Whole Body Conditioners... Your "Aerobic" Quotient

Overall conditioning is essential to health, fitness, and your figure. Such a simple thing as brisk walking is surely one of the easiest, safest, and most convenient ways of getting a whole body workout. You can do it any place at any time. All you need is a good pair of running or walking shoes. Walking is much gentler on your body than running—and just as effective when it comes to burning calories, increasing your heart rate, speeding up your metabolism, and promoting deep breathing. As a bonus, it clears your head, improves concentration, and sharpens creativity.

Effective
Exercise

85

In the past decade or so, we've all been subjected to some rather rigid rules governing aerobic workouts. New research shows that to reap all the benefits of aerobic activity—keep us lean, fit, and healthy; alleviate tension; and lift our spirits—we need not submit to a rigorous marathon routine. Easy does it. Today's more moderate approach to exercise advocates that any significant increase in physical activity will bring you myriad health benefits and extend longevity. There is no need to reach a certain threshold or to do complicated calculations.

Low-intensity aerobics—walking, swimming, bicycling, cross-country skiing, skating—will do wonders to boost circulation of blood and lymph. By doing so, you step up the rate at which cells and tissues absorb oxygen and nutrients. By enhancing lymphatic circulation, you encourage efficient removal of waste products from the tiny spaces between cells. Lymphatic pumping action can increase ten to thirty times its normal rate during a whole-body workout. This, of course, is especially important in conquering cellulite.

Collagen renewal also gets a boost from regular aerobic activity. The rise in skin temperature stimulates the production of collagen, and this results in smoother, younger-looking skin with improved tone and elasticity. Skin thickens with regular exercise, an obvious benefit to counteract the visible signs of premature aging.

Breathing... to Oxygenate and Cleanse
Proper breathing is integral to exercise and vital to health. Whole Body Conditioners certainly promote and regulate deep breathing. As you walk, cycle, swim, or skate, your body adjusts to the activity and you are naturally inclined to inhale deeply and exhale fully. This brings you incalculable benefits, certainly not the least of which is stimulation of lymph flow as breathing is lymph's prime mover. To keep lymph flowing and to make it possible for the lymphatic vessels to carry on their important task of bodily cleansing, we must breathe deeply and often.

Stretching... for Flexibility and Rejuvenation
To develop and maintain flexibility, stretching is essential. This is as important to the average person as it is to the athlete or dancer. We are all born flexible. As we grow older, however, this natural flexibility gradually diminishes, a process we encourage with sedentariness. The more we sit, the faster our muscles and joints lose their full range of motion, making us look and feel older than we are. You will want to include a variety of stretching movements in your daily program, espe-

cially as a "cool down" following any exercise. Think of stretching as a form of "breathing" for your muscles and connective tissue.

When to Exercise
Exercise should never be a chore that you put off until tomorrow or the day after. It should be a pleasant, easy, convenient, and permanent part of your life. A good time to exercise is any time that suits you. The easier it is, the more likely you are to do it. It's a good idea though to exercise at the same time every day, as this assures that it will become a habit— an enjoyable habit that gives you pleasure, satisfaction, and a sense of well-being.

A Final Word to the Exercise-Wise
There is one more thing to keep in mind about exercise. You must be patient. If you are out of shape, you must remember that you did not get this way overnight. All the positive changes that you expect will take place over a period of time. Avoid doing too much in the beginning. Work slowly but surely. If you do too much at first, there's a greater chance of dropping out. It's very often the overly enthusiastic who are the first to quit. Listen to your body. Build up gradually. Stick with it. It will pay off. For sure.

POSTURE: THE PLACE TO START
Good posture uplifts your body and makes you look thinner instantly, and it is a must for good physiology. Poor posture inhibits the flow of oxygen through the body, increases tension, and creates unnecessary aches, pains, and muscle fatigue. It also makes for poor muscle tone, crowds the organs, interferes with proper digestion and elimination, and impedes good circulation.

The secret to good posture is to keep the abdomen pulled in and the rib cage lifted out of the hips. When this is done, everything else falls into place.

The way your body ultimately shapes up depends a lot on good posture or the proper use of your body. So always remember to stand, walk, and sit "tall." It gives you more energy and vitality—and a better outlook on life in general.

Effective Exercise

87

BODY SHAPERS

Reshaping the body involves building muscles in those areas where muscle tissue has slackened. These exercises really work because they target specific muscle groups in stubborn trouble spots with precision and intensity—and in a very short time deliver visible results. Whether you want to maintain an already good figure, or remodel a less than perfect one, these Body Shapers are just what you're looking for. You can slim your thighs, lift your buttocks, flatten your stomach, and even shape your arms in only about twenty minutes a day. By isolating certain muscles, until now neglected or underused, these powerful movements lift and tone without creating bulk. The overall result: a sleeker, slimmer silhouette with less room for cellulite to form.

This Body Shaping program is extremely flexible. Not all the movements need be done in a single session. Although thighs and buttocks should be worked together, abdomen and arms may be worked separately if this is more convenient for you. Of course, if you prefer to do everything at once, that's fine, too. Your own schedule should dictate the timing and the order.

How often? Four or five times a week until you are satisfied with the results. Then three times a week for maintenance.

Body Shaping Pointers

- Focus on form. It is better to do just a few movements correctly than to do a lot of them the wrong way.
- Work muscles in both directions—resisting gravity on the way up and on the way down.
- Go slowly but surely. Never rush through an exercise. If you speed up along the way and use momentum to carry through the movement, chances are you're not working the muscles that the exercise is designed to use.
- Keep movements small and subtle. This is the key to reaping the benefits of any "isolation" exercise, which is what most of these are.
- Aim for slow, controlled motions—avoid jerky ones.
- Keep the muscles being worked "flexed" through the range of movement and tighten some more at peak contraction.
- Throughout the exercises, be sure to keep your abdomen pulled in and do not allow your back to arch.
- Build up gradually. If you haven't exercised in a while, it is best to do just a few repetitions at first to minimize soreness and avoid discouragement.
- Breathe properly throughout. Never hold your breath while exercising. Just breathe normally. Try to take a couple of deep breaths every now and then and exhale forcefully. This will speed up the elimination of waste products, mainly lactic acid, which cause muscle soreness. And, of course, proper breathing encourages better lymph drainage.

WARM UP/LIMBER UP

It's a good idea to limber up with a few movements before a workout, especially if you exercise early in the morning or after a day sitting at a desk. You might also want to include some neck movements (see pages 142–143).

REACHES: Stand with feet shoulder-width apart, stomach pulled in, and rib cage lifted up. Raise your arms and reach up as if to touch the ceiling, first with one arm, then with the other. Keep alternating. Feel the stretch all along the sides of the torso. Repeat 10 times on each side.

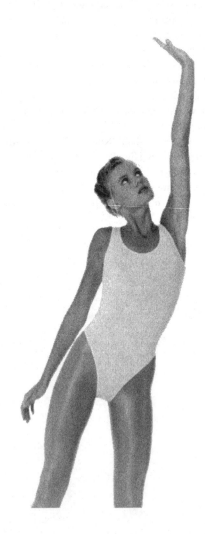

Now, keeping your back straight, bend forward at the waist and reach forward to the opposite side as though you're pushing something away from you. Alternate arm. Repeat 10 times on each side.

While still bending forward at the waist, move your arms in wide semi-circles as if you were swimming; reach as far as you can all the way through. Do other arm. Repeat 10 times alternating arms.

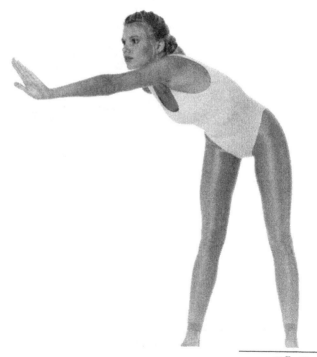

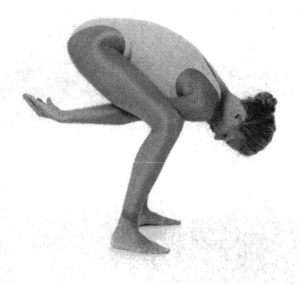

SWING DOWN: Stand with feet shoulder-width apart, rib cage lifted up, and stomach pulled in. Clasp hands overhead. Bend your knees and swing your arms down between your legs. Return to a standing position, swinging your arms back over your head. Do not arch your back. Repeat 10 times.

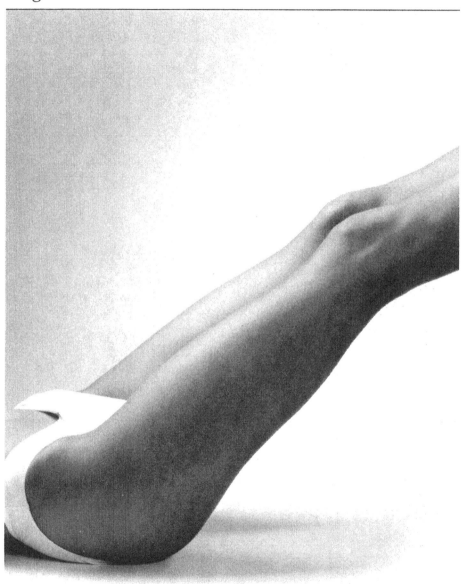

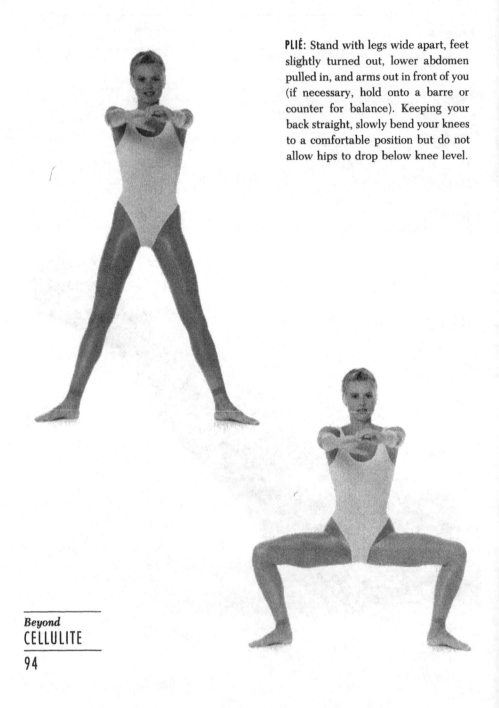

PLIÉ: Stand with legs wide apart, feet slightly turned out, lower abdomen pulled in, and arms out in front of you (if necessary, hold onto a barre or counter for balance). Keeping your back straight, slowly bend your knees to a comfortable position but do not allow hips to drop below knee level.

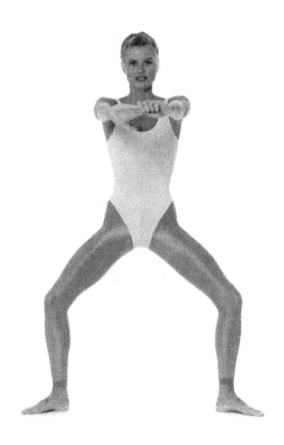

Slowly straighten up partway as shown. Then lower again. Repeat 10 times. Work up to 20.

As your legs get stronger, you can add an extra step: In the deep position on your last repetition, "pulse" 10 times (pulsing means very small movements, in this case up and down, no more than a half-inch in each direction), then hold for 10 counts. Slowly return to a standing position.

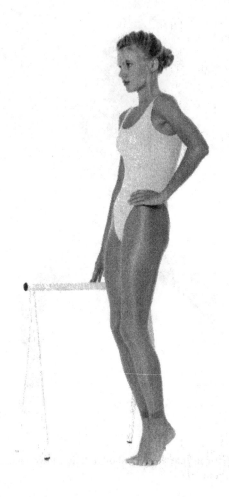

THIGH TONER: Holding onto a barre or counter, stand on the balls of your feet as shown, legs together, and knees slightly bent. Tighten buttocks,

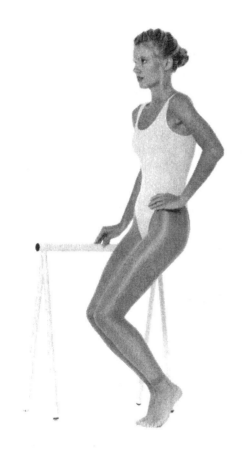

pull stomach in, and slowly lower your body 3 to 5 inches. Hold 3 slow counts. Slowly return to starting position. Repeat 10 times.

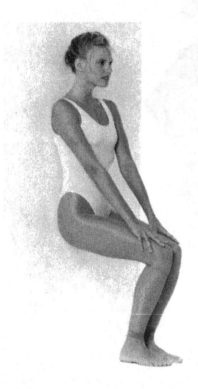

WALL SITTING: Position your body approximately 18 to 24 inches from a wall (preferably a door or a wall with a glossy surface). Lean against wall with a flat back. Now slide down to a sitting position. Knees should be directly over feet. Hold this position to a slow count of 5. Then gently slide back up. Repeat 5 times. Rest as needed.

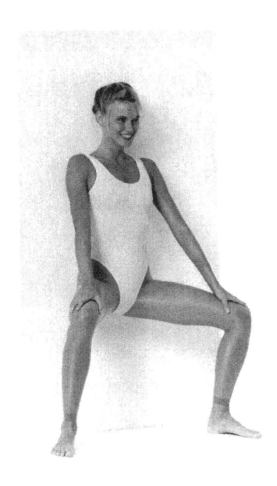

WALL SITTING—SECOND POSITION: Start in the same basic position as above but this time with legs spread wide apart and feet comfortably turned out. Slide down to sitting position. Hold for a slow count of 5. Repeat 5 times. Work up to 10.

Although these two movements appear similar, each works the muscles differently. Therefore, you will want to include both in your program, though perhaps with reduced repetitions in the beginning.

As your muscles get stronger, you may want to increase holding time gradually to 10 to 15 seconds per repetition, adding only a few seconds at a time.

Effective
Exercise

99

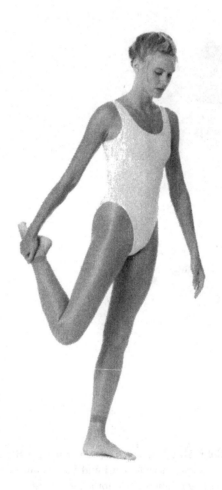

FRONT THIGH STRETCH: While holding onto a support (barre, counter, back of chair), bend one knee slightly, grasp the foot of the other leg and bend it up toward buttocks. Hold 10 counts. Do not arch your back and do not allow the foot to touch your buttocks.

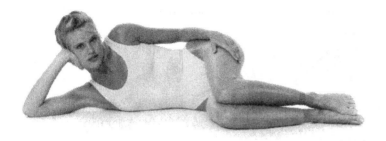

SIDE LEG LIFT: Lie on your right side; bend and draw knees up until the upper thigh is at a 90 degree angle to your torso. Keeping your feet together for stability, raise the upper leg as shown below. Hold one count. Lower. Repeat 5 to 10 times. Raise and lower slowly, and be sure to control motion in both directions. Turn over and do the same while lying on your left side. You may want to make small adjustments in the angle of hip and knee until you feel the maximum pull along the outer hip.

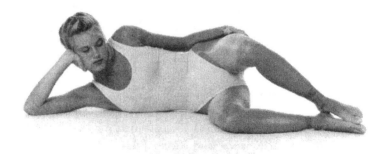

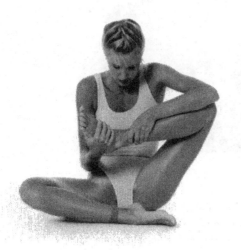

OUTER THIGH STRETCH: Sitting with legs crossed, grab ankle and lift leg toward head as shown. Hold 10 counts. Do other leg.

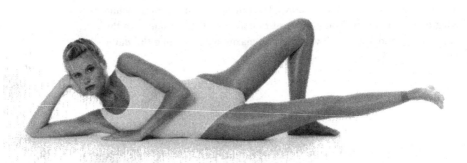

INNER THIGH LIFT: Lie on your right side on your elbow, head resting on hand. Bend your left leg and place your foot flat on the floor as shown. Keeping right leg straight, lift it a few inches off the floor with foot flexed. Hold and slowly lower. Without touching floor, raise leg again. Repeat 10 times. As you gain strength, try pulsing 10 times on your last repetition in raised position. Then hold to a count of 10. Turn over and do the same while lying on your left side. Work up to 2 sets.

Make sure your hip, knee, and foot are in a straight line. Do not lean back. Do not swing or kick your leg up. Concentrate on keeping the under leg firm, and use your inner thigh muscle to lift it. Foot should be flexed with heel leading.

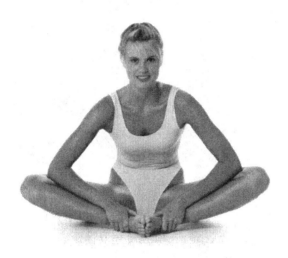

INNER THIGH STRETCH: In seated position as shown, soles of feet together, press knees toward the floor with your elbows. Hold to a count of 10.

Buttocks

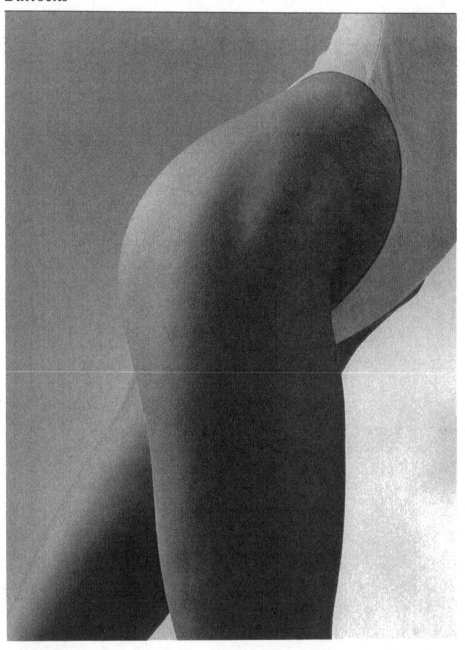

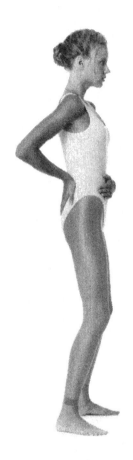 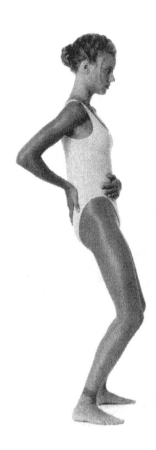

PELVIC TILT: Stand with your feet about 12 inches apart, knees slightly bent, and stomach pulled in. Place one hand on your abdomen the other on your buttock; squeeze buttocks as hard as you can while tilting pelvis upward. Hold for 3 slow counts. Release one count. Repeat 10 times. This is one set. Work up to 2 sets. Stretch buttock between sets by raising one knee chest-high and holding 2 counts, then raise other knee.

The pelvic tilt works the inner thigh as well as the lower abdomen.

Effective
Exercise

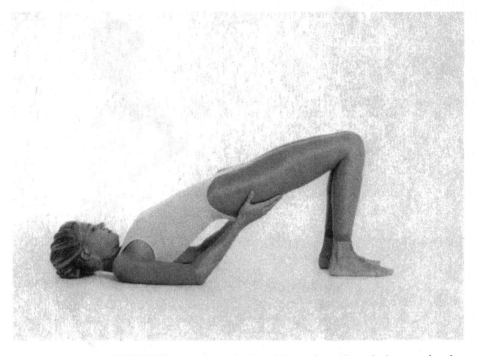

BUTTOCK LIFT: Lie on your back with knees bent, feet a little more than hip distance apart. You may leave your arms on the floor alongside your body or place your hands on your buttocks for movement awareness. Squeeze and tighten your buttock muscles as hard as you can and raise them off the floor as shown. Pause and tighten some more. Lower your hips while keeping muscles flexed, and without touching the floor, go back up. Do not arch your back. Repeat 10 times. Work up to 2 sets. As your muscles get stronger, hold the peak contraction for 3 to 5 counts. Stretch buttocks between sets if necessary by bringing your knees to your chest.

Then place your feet a bit farther apart. Raise your hips as before and bring your knees together while keeping buttock muscles squeezed tight. Open and close knees 10 to 20 times. Resist the motion in both directions by tightening your inner thigh muscles on closing and outer buttocks on opening.

On your last repetition, in the raised position, bring feet hip distance apart, then tilt your pelvis upward while squeezing your gluteus muscles really tight. Pause. Release slightly and repeat 20 times.

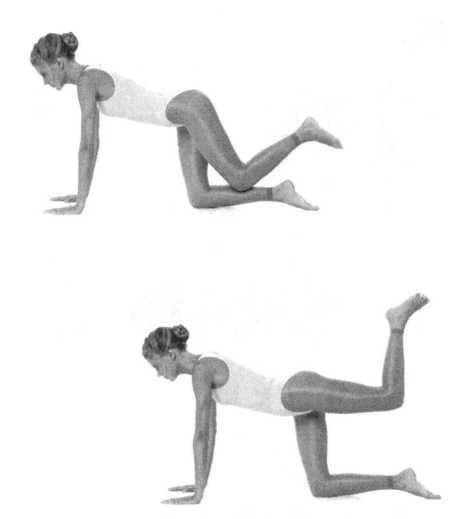

BUTTOCK PRESS: Get down on all fours as shown, or better yet, on bent elbows. Keeping neck aligned with spine and abdominals pulled in, place left knee on right calf. Tightening buttocks, raise left knee to hip level keeping foot flexed. Pause and tighten some more. Then slowly lower to starting position without releasing the grip. Repeat 10 times. Do the same with the other leg.

Effective
Exercise

107

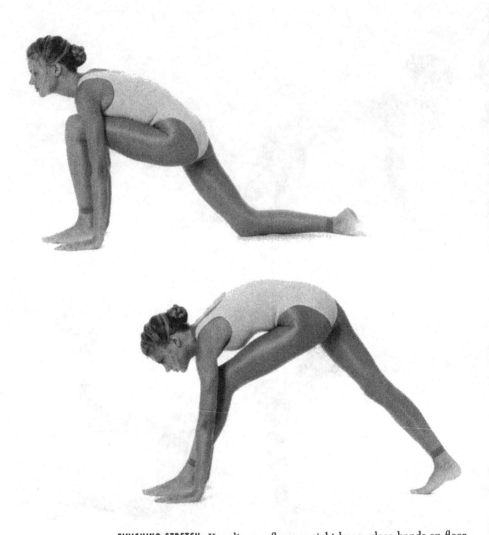

FINISHING STRETCH: Kneeling on floor on right knee, place hands on floor alongside bent leg parallel to calf. Knee should be directly above foot. Slide right leg back as much as you can while keeping front leg stable. Press hips forward. Hold 10 counts. Then try to straighten left knee but only as much as you can; do not strain. Hold 10 counts. Return to starting position by bending right knee and then sliding left leg back into position. Press hips forward. Repeat the whole motion.

This stretches both gluteus and hamstrings.

Stomach

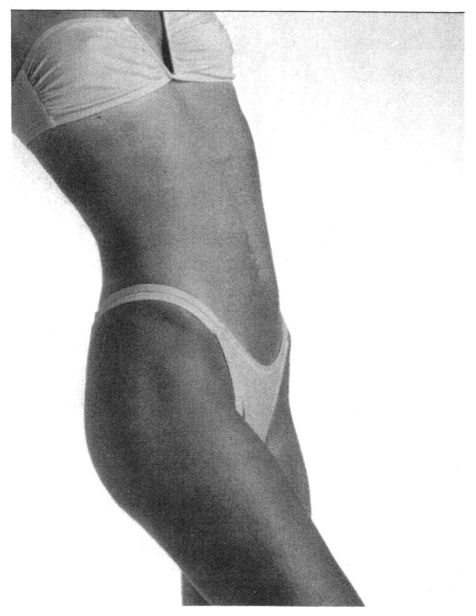

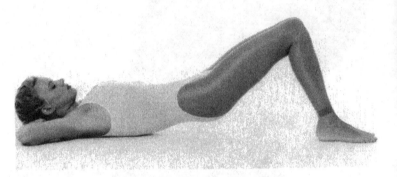

PELVIC CURL: Lie on your back with knees bent and feet shoulder-width apart. Place hands behind your neck or simply leave your arms at your sides. Pull in lower stomach hard and press small of back firmly to the floor lifting buttocks slightly. Hold for 3 to 5 counts. Release. Repeat 10 times. Work up to 30 repetitions.

Be sure only the lower abdominals are used to curl and lift the pelvis. Head can remain on the floor or come up a bit. You may want to exhale fully on your first movement to emphasize that "scooped" feeling.

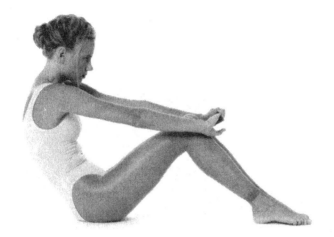

CURL DOWN: Sit on the floor with knees bent and chin tucked in toward your chest. Hold arms out or crossed on chest. Pull in lower abdomen and round lower back. Keep that "hollowed out" feel throughout the exercise. Slowly roll backward, going only as far as you can control. Then, using your stomach muscles, slowly come back up to the starting position keeping back rounded. You may want to exhale as you curl down since this helps you to contract the abdominals further. Take 3 to 5 slow counts to go down, and 3 to 5 slow counts to come back up. Repeat 5 to 10 times.

NOTE: *Do not go all the way down to the floor, as this releases contraction. Contraction must be sustained throughout the movement. It's not important how far you go; the most important thing is to do it right. Be sure the stomach muscles alone are doing all the work in both directions. Keep your movements smooth and slow.*

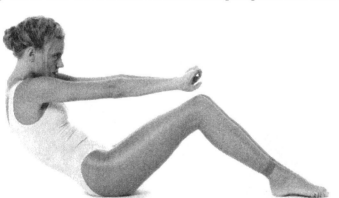

As a variation, instead of just rolling back and curling up, try to pulse 10 times or hold for 10 counts in the farthest position on the roll back. Repeat 5 times. The entire motion should be powered by your abdominals only.

Effective Exercise

111

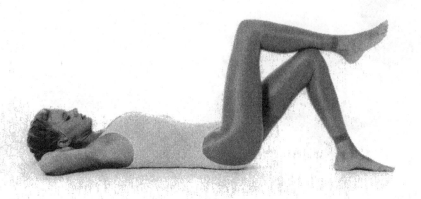

ALL-IN-ONE: Start on the floor as shown, elbows wide, hands behind head, right calf resting on left knee. Pull in lower stomach and flatten small of back against the floor. Using your lower abdominals, raise legs off the floor as shown. Exhale. Lift upper body by contracting upper abdominals.

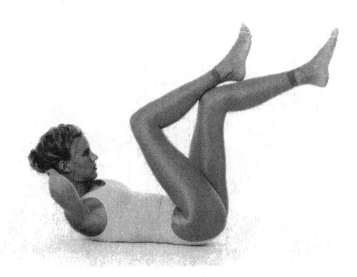

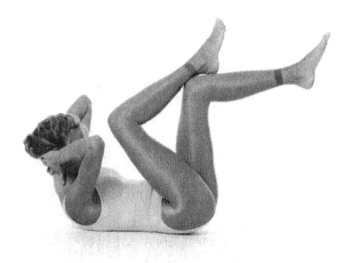

Keep stomach hollowed. Maintaining elevated upper body, exhale again and bring right knee toward right shoulder. Hold 5 counts. Slowly release back to the floor. Start with 5 repetitions and build from there. Repeat on left side.

What makes this exercise special is that it works all stomach muscles: upper, lower, and obliques (sides of waist).

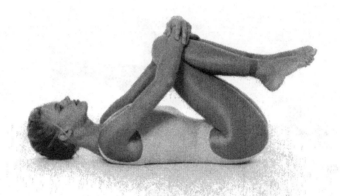

FINISHING STRETCH: Lie flat on your back, bring both knees to your chest, and put one hand on each knee. Bring knees toward your chest without lifting your head. Hold this position for 10 counts. This releases the abdomen and stretches the lower back.

Arms

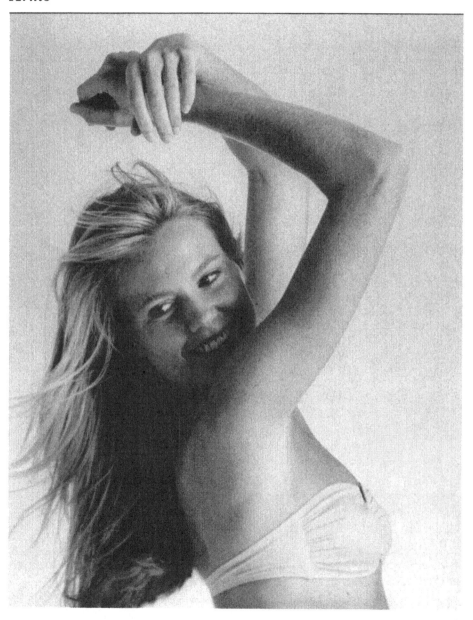

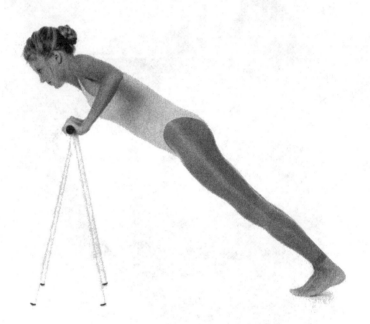

PUSH AWAY: Stand facing support (counter, sofa back). Lean forward; place hands, shoulder-width apart, on edge of support. Keep arms straight, back flat, and stomach pulled in. Slowly bend your elbows and lower body as shown; then, slowly straighten arms and go back up. Repeat 5 to 10 times. Work up to 2 sets.

This works the entire upper body: biceps, triceps, chest, and upper back.

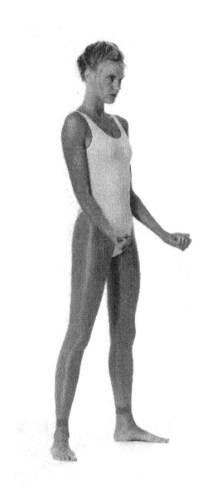 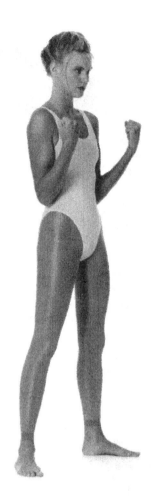

BICEP CURL: Stand with knees slightly bent, feet shoulder-width apart. Hold elbows close to sides throughout the exercise. Curl both arms simultaneously. At peak contraction, pause and tense some more. Lower slowly and repeat. Do 10 times. Work up to 2 sets.

This is best done with free weights or wrist weights. Start with 3 to 5 pounds in each hand and work up. You may also use an alternating motion, raising one arm and then the other. In the absence of weights, clench your fists hard in order to create resistance.

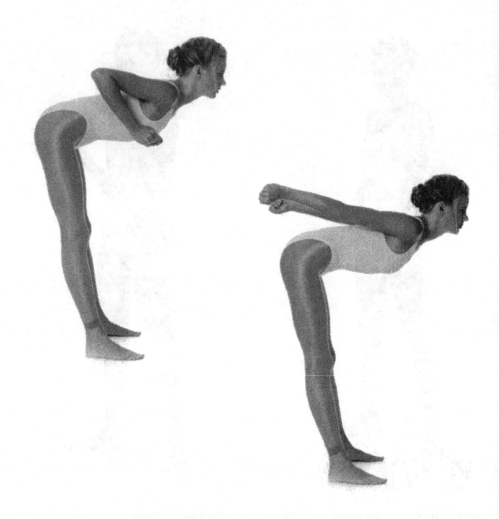

TRICEPS EXTENSION: Bending over with arms flexed at sides, clench fists and extend arms up and back until parallel to floor. Pause for a second and slowly return. Repeat. It is very important to work slowly, controlling the motion in both directions. Repeat 10 times. Work up to 2 sets.

You may wear wrist weights if you like or hold a light dumbbell, lighter than the one used for bicep movements. Control the motion: Do not swing arms.

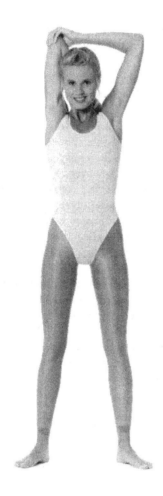

FINISHING STRETCH: With one arm bent behind your head, grasp elbow with other hand. Gently press downward and hold 5 long counts. Do the same with the other arm.

Water Toners

Even though it seems nearly effortless, a vigorous water workout is actually quite powerful and stimulating—with fast, gratifying results. You don't even have to swim a stroke in order to get all the benefits that water has to offer.

The resistance of water is twelve to fourteen times greater than air. This means that your muscles, without the benefit of gravity, are forced to work harder in *every* direction, but you feel far less strain. When you're immersed in water, you "lose" about 90 percent of your weight through the buoyancy factor. No matter what movements you do in water, they'll seem much easier to do than they would on land—certainly less jarring. Studies show that aerobics done in water burn fat more effectively than comparable dry-land routines.

The "massage" benefits of water are unsurpassed. As you move through water, you create forceful "hydroaction," which stimulates the flow of blood and lymph while it tones skin and muscles. Thus, water helps smoothe out the lumps and dimples of cellulite. Your aerobic capacity improves along with overall strength and flexibility. An additional bonus to a nearly perfect workout, water relaxes the mind along with the body, soothing away stress, tension, and worry.

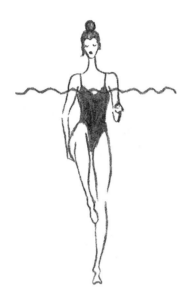

WATER RUNNING: Run in place in chest- or waist-deep water, swinging arms as you would if running on land. Raise your legs high and land flat-footed. Continue for 2 to 3 minutes as a warm-up. For an aerobic workout, run for at least 20 minutes. You may also run/jog across the pool.

For the following exercises, try to spend 2 minutes on each and work up from there.

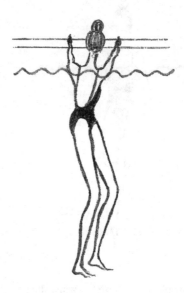

WAIST TWIST: Hold onto the edge of the pool with hands a little more than shoulder-width apart. Without moving your shoulders, twist from side to side as you hop—the motion should only be from the waist down. Be sure to keep your stomach pulled in and your rib cage lifted up.

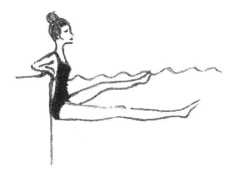

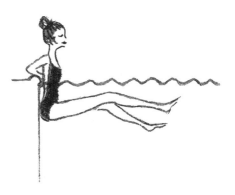

SCISSORS: With your back to the side of the pool, spread arms wide and hold onto pool edge. Bring your legs up. While alternating top and bottom leg in a crossing motion, open and close like a "scissors."

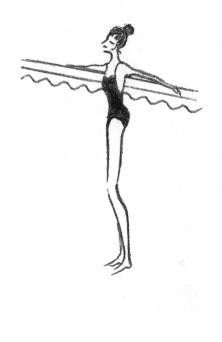

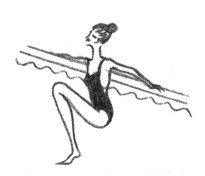

KNEE LIFT: Stand with your back to the side of the pool and the small of your back flat against the pool wall, stomach pulled in, legs extended straight down. Using abdominal muscles, bring knees to chest. Return to starting position and repeat.

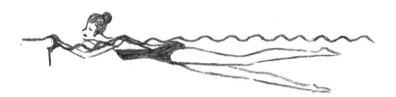

FLUTTER KICK: Face the side of the pool and grip the edge with both hands. Raise your legs and keep them extended directly behind you. Rapidly move your legs in an up-and-down motion. You can also do flutter kicks in motion using a kickboard. Make certain that the movement comes from the gluteal muscles for maximum effectiveness.

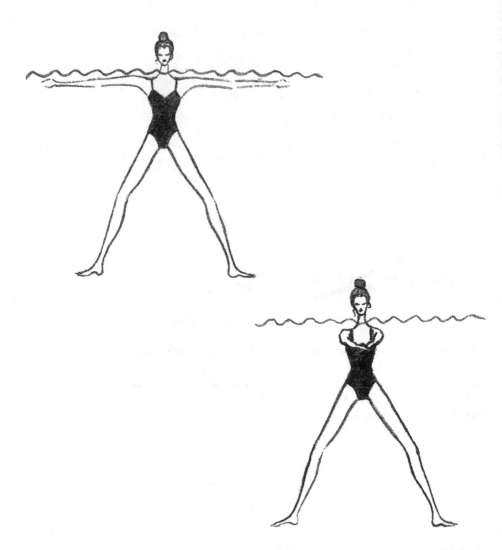

ARM SWEEP: Standing in chest-deep water with feet shoulder-width apart and knees slightly bent, extend your arms out to your sides just below the water's surface. Cup your hands and keep the palms facing forward. Bring your arms forward in a sweeping motion and cross in front of your chest. Then rotating your hands so that the palms are now facing away from each other, sweep your arms back to your sides. Repeat. Make sure that cupped hands always "scoop" water in the direction of movement.

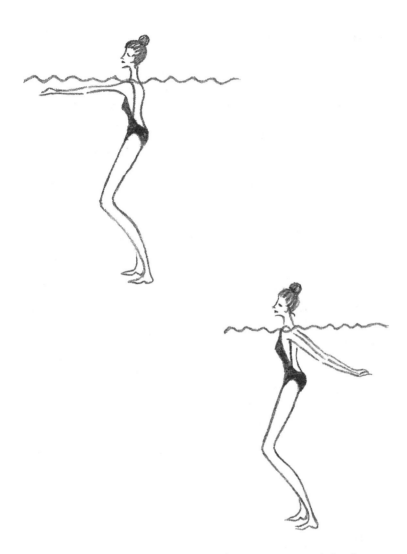

ARM PRESS: Stand in chest-deep water with your arms extended in front of you at surface level. With palms down, lower your arms in a swinging motion all the way back. Rotate hands so that your palms are again facing down and swing arms back to original position. Repeat. Be sure that cupped hands scoop water in the direction of movement.

Effective
Exercise

127

WHOLE BODY CONDITIONERS

Consistency is the key to whole body conditioning. Most experts now seem to agree that instead of a strenuous regimen three times a week, a less intensive and more natural activity such as brisk walking done four to six times a week is preferable. They also point out that you are more likely to stick with a program that is easy to do and convenient. In other words, it's frequency that counts, not intensity.

As for duration, well, that depends upon your level of fitness and the activity itself. Walking is fairly easy to sustain, so you should aim for a minimum of thirty minutes and build up to forty-five. The same applies to bicycling, cross-country skiing, and skating. For a sport like swimming, you may want to start with a shorter span, say twelve to fifteen minutes, and work up to half an hour.

As for "warming up" and "cooling down," there is no special set of exercises. Warming up means using your muscles at a more relaxed pace in the same manner of the actual workout you are about to do. In other words, walking slowly should precede walking briskly, a gentle "crawl" should come before a vigorous swim, and pedaling slowly will prepare you for a bicycle ride. Five to ten minutes of this kind of "warm up" should be adequate for most people. A "cool down" should be simply a gentle and gradual cessation of activity instead of an abrupt halt. Ideally, this should be followed by a few stretching movements.

When choosing a Whole Body Conditioner, keep in mind that whenever you have to go outside to exercise—whether to a pool, a gym, or a park—try to find a location near your home to make exercising as simple and convenient as possible. This will increase your chances of sticking with it. If just getting to your exercise spot becomes too much trouble, you run a much higher risk of dropping out. Consider Whole Body Conditioning a lifetime commitment—a long-term investment in your health, your figure, and your looks.

Walking

Walking is as natural as breathing and should always be an important part of your life for the reasons already discussed. Of course, in order for it to be effective, you must walk fast enough. Essentially, both running and brisk walking burn the same number of calories: 100–110 per mile. The only difference is the time it takes to cover that mile. What really counts, from an aerobic standpoint, is going farther and for a longer period of time rather than speeding up. Four miles per hour—about fifteen minutes per mile—is a good pace. Take long strides. Let your arms swing loosely and naturally; don't hold them tight against your body. Walk "tall" but relaxed.

Walking also just happens to be a perfect activity to include in your daily life. For example, you can walk all the way, or part of the way, to work—if you commute by bus, train, or taxi, you can hop off a stop or two early and walk the rest of the way. Take advantage of your lunch hour to go for a brisk walk, or at least walk to and from the restaurant. Ditto for running errands. When you "walk" your dog, really *walk* him; don't just duck out the door for a minute or two. Also, whenever possible, pass up the elevator or escalator and take the stairs. These may seem like small efforts to make, but they all add up.

In addition to walking, or to add variety to your Whole Body program, here are four sports that are particularly beneficial. Besides keeping you lean, fit, and healthy, they offer tremendous shaping benefits, especially for the lower body.

Bicycling

There is nothing quite like a bike to shape your legs. It gives your thighs that long, lean look if you do it regularly. You don't have to become a cycling buff to get results, nor must you do it for hours on end. Just a nice fifteen- to thirty-minute ride every day during warm weather will give you wonderful results. Depending on where you live, this could be for a good number of months, lasting from early spring right through late fall. Just pick a route around your home to make it convenient. Try to avoid heavy traffic—for the obvious dangers and also because breathing all those fumes is not healthy.

To get maximum results from your bicycle, be sure to adjust the seat height. The correct position is one that allows your legs to be almost fully straight when the pedals are down; there should be no more than a slight bend in the knee. Otherwise, you get robbed of some of the shaping benefits. A full range of motion is very important to avoid developing bulky muscles and to achieve that long, sinuous look. You can also increase resistance for faster results.

Swimming

Regular swimming can do wonders for your health, your head-to-toe fitness, and your looks. The resistance of water forces your muscles to work hard, but the comfort level of this medium makes the workout seem nearly effortless. Cold water also stimulates the redistribution of fatty tissue for overall insulation. And, of course, vigorous swimming promotes fat loss by burning calories rapidly and efficiently.

Because the body is level in swimming, there are no pressure points anywhere. There is no tension. If you watch a good swimmer in motion, you will see long, smooth, powerful strokes that allow the body to glide through the water. The movements are rhythmic and fluid. The breathing is regular and deep.

Swimming is an especially effective cellulite eradicator. It conditions practically every muscle of the body and gets the lymph flowing rapidly and evenly. The powerful massage action of the water also improves skin tone, making it remarkably firm, smooth, and sleek. You rarely see a good swimmer with lumpy thighs. Even at an advanced age, a woman who swims regularly has young-looking and well-toned skin. There are no dimples. There is no sagging.

So, if you're a good swimmer, by all means start to swim regularly. If you're not good at this sport but like the water, you might want to investigate the many options for adult swim lessons at a local "Y" or health club. You might also look into water exercise classes, sometimes called "aqua aerobics." These have become quite popular and for good reasons: They're effective, enjoyable, and a great alternative for those who do not swim.

Cross-Country Skiing

This is a truly remarkable sport. And so very pleasant. Like swimming, it works the entire body—the arms are as active as the legs. Many muscle groups get involved in the steady, rhythmic motion of this sport.

The friction of the skis against the snow has an extraordinarily calming effect. Anxiety is left behind as you enter the snowy meadows and the quiet country lanes. Also, this is a sport that anyone can practice. If you ski on fairly flat terrain, no special skill is required. And the risks of injury are very low.

You can increase the challenge of this sport simply by heading for more hilly trails. Terrain choices are varied and entirely your own. Although it is not absolutely necessary, you may want to gain your introduction to this sport through a qualified instructor or a friend who is good at it. One more advantage: The equipment is relatively inexpensive and no special clothing is required.

Skating

Skating provides quite an effective way to get a lower-body workout. The motion of "pushing off" from the inside edge of one skate onto the other skate, when executed properly, is a real leg-shaper as it works all the muscles from calf to upper thigh. This activity encourages regular, deep breathing, a superb benefit especially when ice-skating outdoors in the frosty air of winter. It also works two parts of the body more directly than other sports do. Since the gluteal muscles are brought into the motion, the upper thigh and buttocks will be lifted and tightened. Also, the inner thigh, one of those hard-to-reach areas, will be firmed and strengthened by the "gripping" motion that controls gliding and balance. If you watch figure skaters in competition, you cannot help but notice their powerful yet gracefully formed legs.

Roller skating will also give you shape and contour—and it's great fun, too. If you take up ice skating during the colder months, you can easily switch to roller-blading in spring and summer. This relatively new sport is quickly gaining popularity from coast to coast. Conventional roller-skating is also a fine way to continue your workout year-round.

Indoor Versions

Just as cycling can be done indoors as well as walking on a treadmill, so can cross-country skiing. Though you can derive the same benefits, the indoor versions have advantages and disadvantages. The scenery is certainly not the same and you don't get the benefit of fresh air. On the other hand, you can get your exercise rain or shine, day or night. So I guess you must take the pros and cons into consideration, and perhaps find a happy medium by combining the real thing with the indoor version.

Stretching

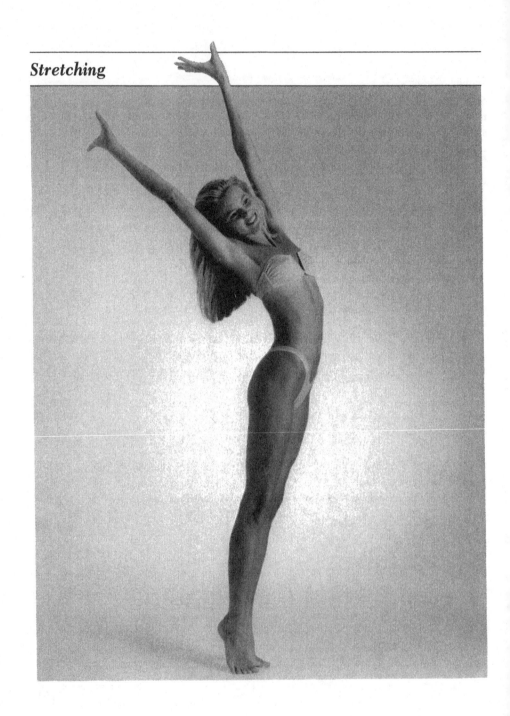

Stretching is a must for everyone regardless of age or flexibility. For best results, you should include a variety of stretching exercises in your daily program. You can do the entire routine outlined here or select a few movements according to your needs.

Here are some of the benefits you will reap from stretching:

- Stretching stimulates the circulation of blood and lymph. By stretching your body regularly, you will keep lymph flowing more freely.
- Stretching after a workout helps muscles recuperate by restoring those shortened by exercise back to their resting length.
- Stretching relaxes muscles and helps alleviate the various aches caused by stress and tension.
- Stretching slows down or prevents the gradual stiffening associated with the aging process. The attributes of youth, flexibility and elasticity, are improved, maintained, or restored.
- Muscles that are stretched regularly keep their elastic quality, have better blood flow, and receive nourishment more efficiently.
- Stretching is an effective means of reducing tension as it relaxes the mind while it tones the body.
- Stretching makes you feel tall, lean, and lithe. It improves your posture by conditioning smooth, elongated muscles.

Some Stretching Pointers:

- Always stretch within your own limits. This should be a pleasant, relaxing experience. If it hurts, you have stretched too far.
- Always do a "holding" stretch—never bounce.
- An ideal time to stretch is right after a workout, a brisk walk, or some other form of aerobics. Also, since stretching relieves muscle tension, it can be used any time to make you feel better all over.
- Always breathe while stretching. The point to remember is neither to hold your breath nor to overbreathe. It is best to breathe normally and smoothly. In between stretches, breathe in deeply and exhale fully.

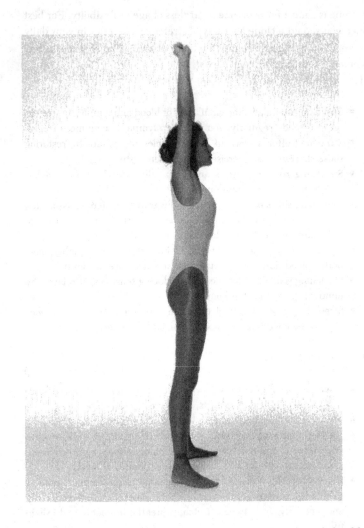

1: Bring your arms overhead and stretch, lifting rib cage and shoulders. Hold 5 counts.

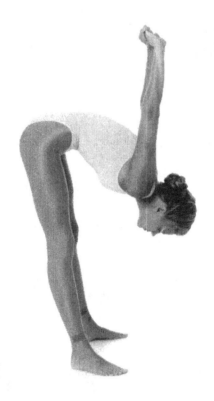

2: Now bring your arms behind your back, clasp hands, pull stomach in, and bend forward at the waist, go only as far down as you can. Hold to a slow count of 15.

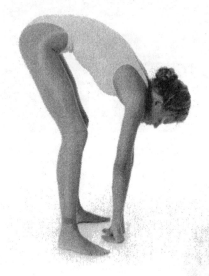

3: Bending your knees, bring your hands to the floor.

3-A: Straighten your knees only as much as you can. Hold 15 counts. Slowly come back up, uncurling the spine one verte-brae at a time.

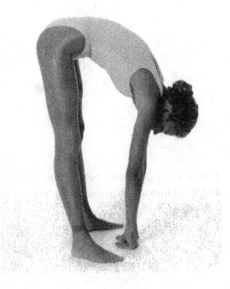

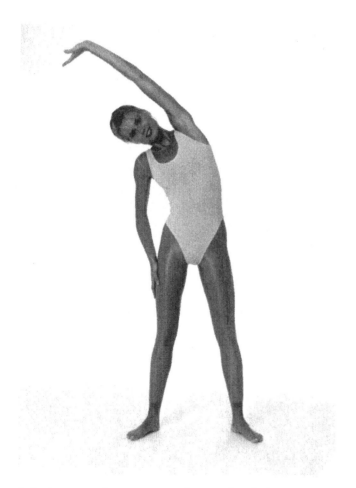

4: Again in a standing position, with stomach pulled in and rib cage lifted up, place your right hand on upper right thigh, and bring your left arm over your head. Stretch all the way to the right side as if to push a wall. Hold 15 counts. Slowly return to the standing position and do the other side.

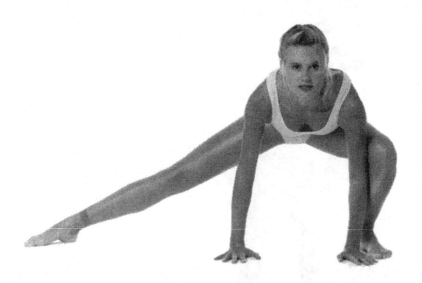

5: Spread legs wide apart, place hands on floor. Slide your right leg out to the side as you bend your left knee as shown. Feel the stretch all along the inner thigh. Hold 10 to 15 counts. Switch legs and do the other side. Be sure to keep your feet flat on the floor.

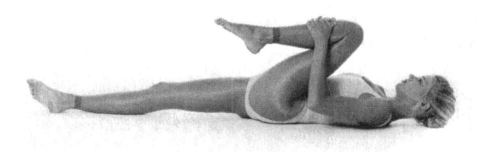

6: Lying on your back, bring your right knee to your chest. Hold for 5 counts.

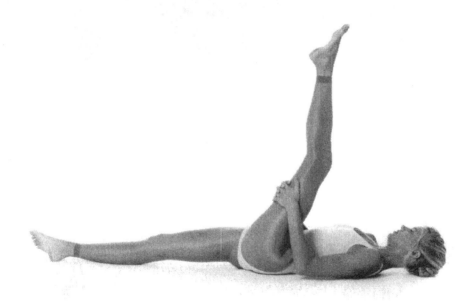

6-A: Now straighten your right leg only as far as is comfortable and try to bring it toward you. Hold for 10 to 15 counts. Slowly lower leg. Do the same with the left leg.

Effective
Exercise

139

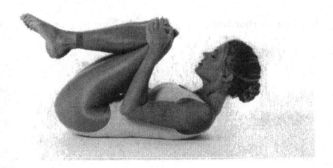

7: Lying on your back, bring both knees to your chest. Hug your knees and bring your head toward them. Hold for 10 to 15 counts.

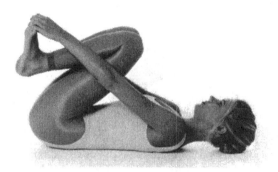

8: Lying on your back, bring both knees to your chest and grasp your toes.

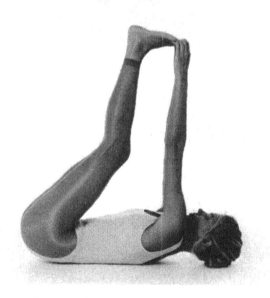

8-A: Gently straighten your knees only as far as you can. Hold for 10 to 15 counts.

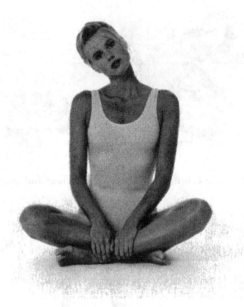

9: While sitting or standing, look straight ahead, press head toward one shoulder. Hold for 5 counts. Lift head and then bend toward other shoulder. Repeat twice.

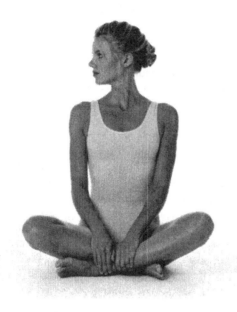

10: While sitting or standing, look straight ahead, turn your head to one side and look over your shoulder. Hold for 5 counts. Slowly return your head to its original position, then turn it to the other side and hold. Repeat twice.

At the end of your stretching routine, take several deep breaths.

BREATHING

Each of us takes about 20,000 breaths a day, yet there is no bodily function that gets less of our conscious attention than breathing. We rarely think about it at all—until it is impaired or threatened in some way. But there are tremendous benefits to be derived from proper breathing.

The effect of breathing on lymph drainage is one physiological fact hardly ever mentioned. Everyone knows that breathing brings oxygen to cells and releases carbon dioxide, but it does more than that. Breathing is responsible for removing cellular wastes and toxins that accumulate in tissue spaces as a result of cell metabolism. It does this through its direct action on the movement of lymph.

You will recall that the lymph, our secondary circulation, has no pumping mechanism to power its flow. It relies, for the most part, on muscle contraction and the suction of breathing for its circulation. The diaphragm, the muscle that separates the thorax from the abdomen, is our most important lymphatic "pump." During deep breathing, the movements of the diaphragm allow the lymph to flow normally. This assistance is made possible by the changes of pressure in the thoracic and abdominal cavities. During inspiration, the lymphatic vessels are expanded in the thorax and compressed in the abdomen as a result of the changes in pressure. During expiration, the effects are reversed as the pressure swings in the opposite direction.

When the vessels are enlarged, more lymph enters them from below. When they are compressed, lymph is forced upward. This accessory "pumping" action with every respiration considerably aids the flow of lymph in the lower limbs. When this flow is sluggish, a stagnation of the interstitial fluid occurs. In the hips and thighs, this excess of interstitial fluid encourages the formation of cellulite.

Such a simple thing as conscious breathing can help tremendously to keep the body free of wastes and toxins. Most of us use only about half our full breathing potential. Therefore, we expel only about half the accumulated waste products, and we benefit from only half the oxygen we could otherwise have in our systems. With a little concentration on breathing, we can increase the benefits not only to the lymph but to all the cells of the body. Benefits here include youthful-looking skin, increased vitality, calmer emotions, and clearer thinking.

Some Breathing Exercises

Here are two very effective techniques. For the first one, called the "Replenishing Breath," breathe in the following pattern: inhale for a count of 4, hold for a count of 4, exhale for a count of 4. This is one cycle. Repeat: in 4, hold 4, out 4. Work up to 10 cycles.

Aim for two or three sessions of 10 cycles a day, preferably outdoors, where you are surrounded by fresh, clean air. Also, as you progress with deep-breathing techniques, you'll want to incorporate them with your Whole Body Conditioners such as walking—or at the end of a refreshing swim.

After you have mastered the 4-4-4 Replenishing Breath, you may want to increase your capacity for deep breathing with the 4-4-8 (inhale 4, hold 4, exhale 8). In time, you will move on to an advanced pattern of 4-8-12 (inhale 4, hold 8, exhale 12).

Another technique that you will want to incorporate into your program comes from yoga and is called the "Cleansing Breath." This is similar to the other technique except that the exhalation pattern is more deliberate and forceful. You inhale deeply through your nostrils and audibly release the breath little by little through pursed lips. The goal here is to release the breath as thoroughly as possible and from way down in the abdomen, forcing out as many wastes as you can in short bursts.

The Cleansing Breath makes you more aware of the exhalation process while improving overall breathing capacity and strengthening abdominal muscles. At first, you should be able to manage at least ten releasing bursts per breath. Then breathe normally a couple of moments and repeat the cycle a few times. After a while, you will probably reach twelve or more purifying exhalations per breath. Try to do this exercise at least twice a day.

Deep-breathing techniques are wonderfully invigorating yet supremely relaxing. In addition to your regular sessions, you may want to use the Replenishing Breath and/or the Cleansing Breath whenever you feel sluggish or unsettled. And at night, right before bedtime, you may wish to breathe deeply to relax your entire body. Just stand near an open window or on a terrace and inhale the clear night air.

There are a few things to keep in mind when practicing breathing techniques. You should never strain. Start with a low count and gradually build up as you develop better lung capacity. In the beginning, you should go easy. Like stretching, there is no particular goal to reach here; just do the exercises naturally and comfortably. Never exceed your own capacity—and never to the point of lightheadedness.

GRAVITY... AND HOW TO FIGHT IT

With time, gravity takes its toll, and the entire body is affected. This is especially true if muscles are not kept in top shape so they can hold everything up. We've all noticed how we seem to get thicker, bulkier, and wider with time even without putting on extra weight. Skin begins to sag. If muscles do not have enough tone, they, too, begin to droop—and they take everything down with them.

The best protection against the relentless pull of gravity, then, is good muscles—toned, firm, tight, and strong. The Body Shapers, when performed regularly, will certainly help to achieve this condition. Many of the Whole Body Conditioners will also keep muscles in prime shape.

And then there are those "extra" things we can do to counteract gravity. A slantboard is particularly effective because it's easy to use, and it allows for long, sustained periods of reversal. Another good method is the shoulder stand: Lie on your back and bring your knees to your chest, raise your hips off the floor, supporting your back with your hands, and slowly straighten your legs.

In addition to the slantboard there is other equipment designed to reverse the effects of gravity. Inversion boots and tables are quite effective, but they may not be suitable for everyone. If you decide to use one of these, be certain to follow the manufacturer's instructions carefully. It's also a good idea to have someone nearby in case a "rescue" is warranted.

By "reversing" the flow of fluids in the body—blood and lymph—you can increase nourishment of cells and accelerate the removal of wastes. Oxygenation to the brain is improved, which results in clearer thinking, better memory function, and increased serenity. Sagging or prolapsed organs can be coaxed back to their proper position. Facial lines and sagging contours can be minimized. Better blood flow means better skin tone along with a healthier complexion and scalp. Also, you can combat a water retention problem by reversing gravity's tug. All in all, these various methods have a remarkable, rejuvenating effect on the entire body.

The Slantboard

This is truly a wonderful invention and so sublimely simple. Of all the methods of gravity reversal, the slantboard is the real classic and the favorite of many people. It has been said that a fifteen-minute recline on a slantboard provides the equivalent restfulness of one hour's sleep. This is a perfect way to relax after a full day of work—and a wonderfully restorative prelude to an evening out.

The inclined position is excellent for deep diaphragmatic breathing. To get maximum benefits, rest your hands on the abdomen and breathe deeply; as you exhale, press gently. You can improve lymphatic circulation and drainage tremendously with this technique.

Two 15-minute sessions a day are ideal. You will want to work toward this goal gradually—just a few minutes at a time, especially if it feels uncomfortable in any way. Also, remember to rise slowly from the board to prevent dizziness.

7

Skin Workout

WHY THE SKIN MUST BE KEPT ACTIVE

ike muscles, the skin must also be kept active through a form of "exercise" or workout. In Europe, people have understood for years the value of caring for the skin in this way. Certain techniques, which will be fully explained and demonstrated in this chapter, have a dramatic and wonderful effect not only on surface skin but on the tissue that lies directly beneath it. Long-standing European traditions, *skin brushing* and *self-massage*, when practiced regularly, are more than beauty aids. They are great enhancers of health, vitality, and overall fitness. Our total "Skin Workout" is designed to produce results that are far more than skin deep.

Brushing and massage can work wonders to influence the layer of subcutaneous tissue where cellulite is lodged. Your skin will come alive with the polished glow of youthful vitality, and other things will be happening, too. These methods will stimulate microcirculation, speed up lymph drainage, reduce puffiness, and smooth out the lumps and bumps. You will look and feel briskly rejuvenated in the process.

By stimulating the outermost layer of skin, we can directly alter connective tissue. By working from the "outside," we affect the "inside." This is an integral part of our Anti-Cellulite Strategy and another way of

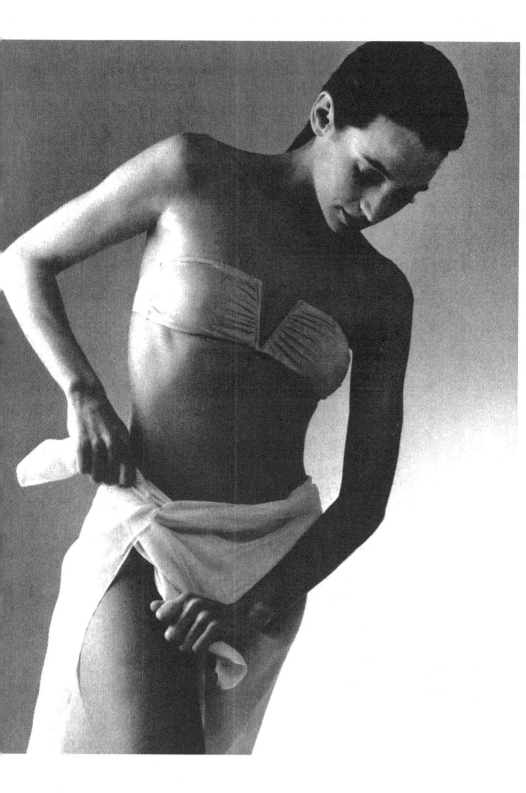

improving overall physiology. In conjunction with proper eating habits, exercise, and stress management, these techniques will greatly accelerate the elimination of cellulite.

Brushing and massage both serve to break up the viscous material or congestion of cellulite into a more fluid form. The lymphatic system can then function with renewed efficiency to process this fluid and keep it flowing more evenly. This is a very gentle yet powerful way of cleansing the tiny tissue spaces of accumulated wastes so that they can be whisked away by the bloodstream and the lymph.

Perhaps, at this point, it is necessary to clear up a general misconception about skin brushing and massage. By themselves, these techniques cannot make us lose weight nor will they burn up fat in targeted areas. Instead, they encourage the body to work more efficiently, and if weight loss is desirable, it can be enhanced with these practices. When the body functions at its best, all systems become more responsive.

SKIN TALK: A FEW WORDS ABOUT SKIN

The skin is the body's largest organ of elimination. So effective is it in clearing the body of wastes that it is often called the "third kidney." Without realizing it and without feeling it, we eliminate up to a pound of wastes every day through the skin. Much of this occurs through imperceptible perspiration.

Hundreds of thousands of very tiny sweat glands serve not only to regulate body temperature but to expel impurities. An estimated 2 million pores are really conduits of elimination that act around the clock to detoxify the body. When these pores are clogged or inactive, a tremendous burden is placed on the other organs of elimination.

Besides serving as a major purifying organ, the skin performs a multiplicity of functions. It "breathes" by drawing oxygen from the air and exhaling carbon dioxide. It is capable of absorbing certain vitamins, minerals, and proteins with which it comes in contact, and by a mysterious chemical process, it manufactures Vitamin D. Obviously, the skin serves as a shield to protect bones, muscles, and organs from invasion by bacteria and other harmful substances. And it holds everything together in one neat wrapper. It even supplies its own conditioner or moisturizer with the production of sebum. There is no replacement or substitute for vital living skin.

The vast network of capillaries under the skin is connected with larger veins. The highest concentration of lymphatic vessels lies in this same tissue layer. So the way we treat the skin has benefits and consequences far deeper than we may realize at first.

WHAT SKIN BRUSHING AND SELF-MASSAGE CAN DO
Faithful practice of these methods will:

- Greatly improve circulation in the capillaries. One of our goals is to improve microcirculation, and skin brushing accomplishes this by stimulating activity in these tiny vessels.
- Improve exchanges between cells and interstitial fluid. This means that the process of cell nourishment and cell renewal will be greatly stepped up.
- Speed up the removal of cellular wastes from the spaces between cells. This will go a long way toward alleviating the congestion in the internal environment.
- Greatly improve lymphatic flow. The lymph, you will recall, circulates slowly and against gravity. We can give it a boost by encouraging its flow toward the lymph nodes or filtering stations. This is crucial in conquering the lumps and bumps.
- Help flush excess water from tissues and thus reduce the tendency toward puffiness and bloating.
- Hasten tissue healing and repair. Keep in mind that healthy, firm tissue depends upon efficient cell renewal and repair.
- Relax muscles and cleanse them of wastes and impurities. Good muscle tone depends upon healthy muscles.
- Render connective tissue more supple and malleable. Collagen and elastin, the fibers that support skin, will also benefit through accelerated renewal and thus minimize premature aging.
- Allow the skin to breathe more freely by opening the pores. This will also improve the functioning of other organs by relieving some of the burden placed on them by skin that is clogged and sluggish.
- Improve the texture and quality of the skin by stimulating the hormone and oil-producing glands.
- Protect the body against illness by improving the lymphatic system. Since the lymph is integral to the body's immune system, better lymph flow will lead naturally to a higher level of immunity. Many people who practice daily skin brushing actually report fewer common ailments such as headaches, colds, and flu symptoms.

Dry Skin Brushing: How to Do It

This is best accomplished with a natural bristle brush that has a long detachable handle. You will find a selection of these brushes at health food stores and many pharmacies.

Begin by standing in a comfortable position. Place one foot on a higher surface, such as the edge of the bathtub or a bed. Start by brushing the soles of the feet from toes to heel. Proceed to the top of the foot and move upward: calves, thighs, buttocks. Give extra attention to the skin between knees and waist, going over the cellulite areas several times, alternating circular motions with long sweeping motions. The direction of brushing should always be from the extremities toward the lymph node sites in the groin, abdomen, and armpits. Now do the upper body: palms of hands, backs of hands, and arms—sweeping toward the armpits. Next, do your shoulders and back (you might need the long handle now), bringing the motions around the torso toward the abdomen. For the front of your torso, an especially sensitive area, gently move downward from chest to abdomen. Finish with gentle circular motions in the abdominal and groin area. Be sure to cover each part of the body a few times with long sweeping strokes and/or circular motions.

Brushing should be firm and vigorous but not overly so. You may achieve a rosy glow, but do not brush until your skin is red or irritated. The entire procedure should take only three to five minutes.

Some dry skin brushing pointers are:

- The best times to brush are morning and before bedtime. Some people like to follow brushing with a shower, bath, or rubdown with a damp sponge.
- Depending upon the sensitivity of your skin, you may want to start with a softer brush (but not too soft) and later on, after your skin is accustomed to brushing, use a firmer model.
- You should have your very own brush, just as you have your own toothbrush, reserved for your personal use.
- Every few weeks or so, you will want to clean your brush with mild soap and water. Just let it dry naturally—in the sun or a warm room.
- Avoid brushing areas of the skin that are irritated or bruised.
- Do not brush damp or wet skin as this may cause stretching and sagging. Always use a dry brush on dry skin.

Self-Massage: How to Do It

Massage is a natural complement to skin brushing. With this technique we further work on the areas of the body affected by cellulite to tone and smooth connective tissue. The simplest way to practice self-massage is to include it with a bath or shower.

Use soapy water to facilitate the movements of deep stroking and kneading. Body lotion also makes it easier to massage, and you may want to repeat the motions after your bath or shower as you apply an emollient.

Place your leg on the side of the bathtub or on a stool to relax muscles. The motions for self-massage are kneading and deep-stroking. Always work upward, from knees to buttocks, covering the entire area once or twice. With the entire hand, lift and squeeze, just as if you were working with modeling clay or dough. For the thighs, you might also include a wringing motion in which you rest both hands around the area and twist back and forth in opposite directions. To concentrate on buttocks and upper thighs, you may use both hands, one on each side, working simultaneously in kneading motions. This entire procedure should take only a few minutes. Always finish your massage with deep upward stroking.

Massage should not be in any way traumatic. Under no circumstances should there be pain or bruises. But don't be too gentle either—a mere caress does not accomplish much. Pressure should be firm and purposeful. If you have varicose veins or broken capillaries, or if your circulation is especially poor, use a little extra caution.

Until your cellulite problem is under control, you will want to use self-massage techniques every day for a few minutes at a time. Later, you may wish to switch to a "maintenance" schedule of twice a week.

What About All Those Anti-Cellulite Creams?

If you want to use those to facilitate your massage movements as well as condition and moisturize your skin, that's okay. But don't count on products alone to solve your problem. They won't. In fact, the most reputable firms strongly recommend in their literature that you follow a sensible diet and exercise program along with their product. Beware of suspicious brands with extravagant claims. The more miraculous, the less likely they are to do anything for you. Bear in mind what I've said earlier in this book: To this day, there are no miracle cures. Cellulite can only be treated effectively from the inside out with a total approach. After having read this far, this should make more sense to you than ever.

A Few More Suggestions for Massaging the Body

There is no need to confine massage to the techniques described above. Water, and especially seawater with its long history of healing the body, is Nature's own instrument of massage. But you don't have to wait for your next visit to the seashore to indulge in the various forms of hydromassage.

Swimming, of course, affords one of the best opportunities for a powerful, overall water massage. Any time you are near water, you can actively or even passively avail yourself of its stimulating benefits. In a swimming pool, spend a few extra minutes allowing the jets to massage your hips and thighs. The same holds for a whirlpool or Jacuzzi—just position yourself for maximum stimulation of cellulite-prone areas, and include the soles of the feet, to promote better lymphatic circulation.

At the ocean, of course, you are in a veritable natural spa. The rich waters here create an invigorating massage milieu—and one of the most pleasant ways to get a body rub. Sea algae has long been revered for its properties of healing the body and dissolving cellulite lumps. Just stand or sit along the shoreline and allow the waves to wash or break against your lower body. Rub a little sand on your feet and legs—and watch your skin get polished to a satiny finish.

Breathe the sea air deeply for its cleansing properties. Surf, sand, and salty air are excellent conditioners, and if you have ever spent a season or even a few weeks at the shore, you've probably noticed the wonderful changes in your skin. Its smooth and even texture at the end of your vacation was not due to tanning alone but to the sea's atmosphere. Your whole body breathes and drinks in the healthy benefits.

AIR BATHS

By all means, treat yourself to an "air bath" whenever possible. This is a simple and natural way to expose your skin to the myriad benefits of oxygen. In today's lifestyle, most of us spend too much time in artificial environments with the drying effects of heating and air-conditioning. On top of that, clothing often prevents the body from breathing adequately. Proper oxygenation of the skin is essential.

Frequent, all-over exposure to fresh air will result in improved skin tone, finer texture, and better coloration. When possible, take off all your clothes and allow the life-giving fresh air to circulate all around you.

When at home, slip into loose-fitting garments made from natural

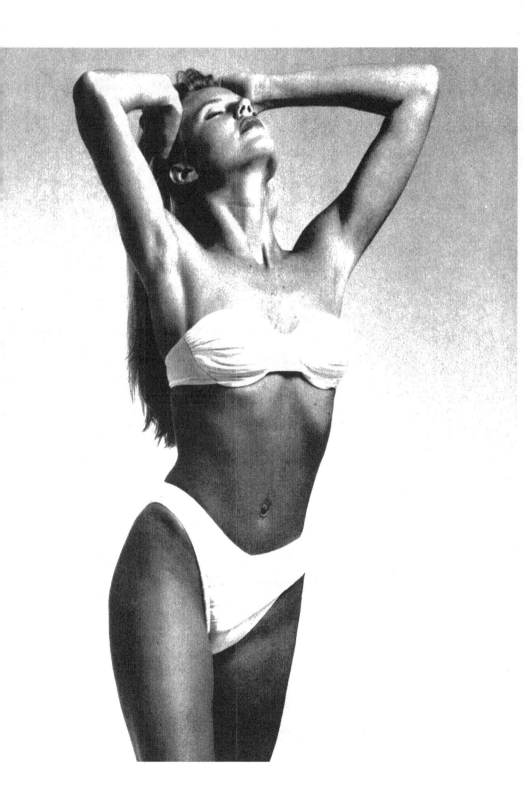

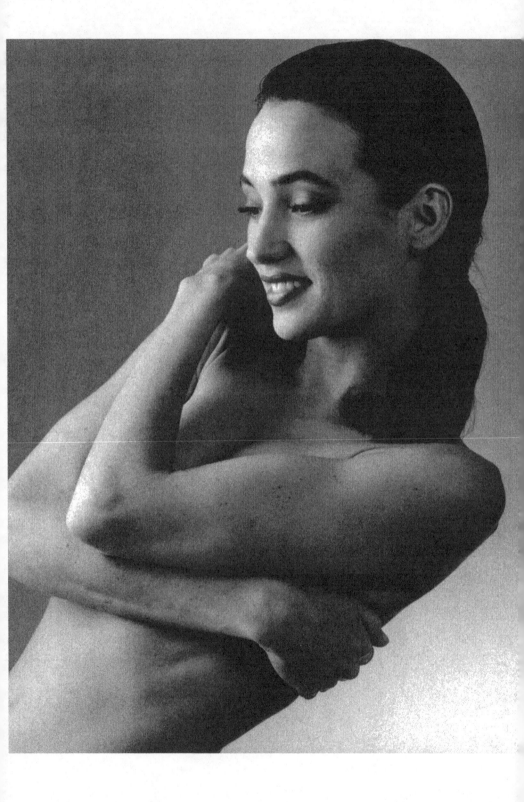

fibers. In fact, it's a good idea to choose cotton, silk, linen, and wool for all your clothing. These fabrics are more in harmony with the body and allow it to breathe freely. Natural fibers keep you cool in summer and warm in winter—whereas synthetic ones are always at odds with the temperature, feeling hot in summer and cold against your skin in winter.

AVOID PROLONGED EXPOSURE TO THE SUN

Avoid sunbathing. As you surely know by now, it is one of the worst, most damaging things you can do to your skin. And one that you can control almost totally.

Although a tan may be flattering to many of us, it is simply not worth the many risks. At worst, overexposure to the sun's rays may lead to skin cancer. At the very least, and perhaps of more immediate concern, such exposure causes premature aging by altering the skin's support system. And while a tan lasts only a short while, the devastating effects remain with you for a lifetime.

You can still enjoy nice color and a healthy glow naturally and without damage if you follow a few simple suggestions. By exposing as much skin as possible to fresh air, you will accomplish this. As soon as weather permits, you can change into shorts, T-shirts, and tank tops. When at the beach or pool, sit under a protective umbrella or in the shade. When boating, always wear protective clothing to shield yourself from sun and wind.

If you still wish to bask in the sun, and there is no doubt that this is a pleasant and sensual experience, try to restrict this activity to early morning (before ten o'clock) and late afternoon (after four o'clock). And always use a good sunscreen.

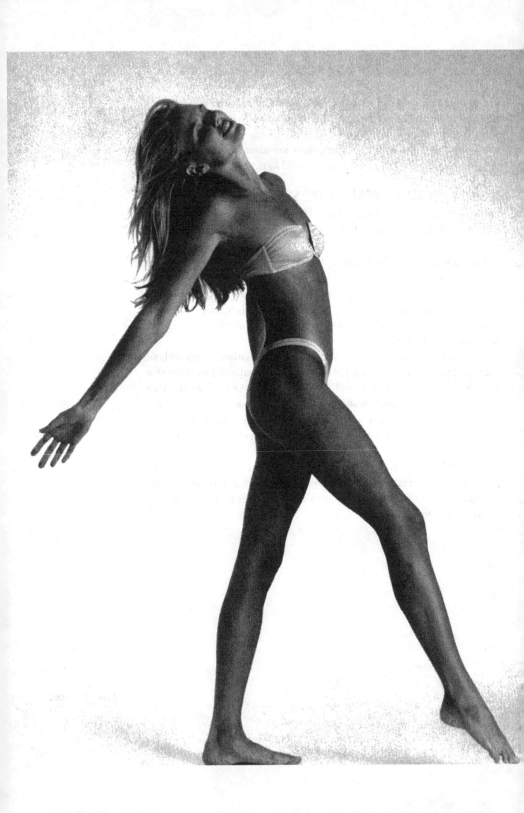

SOME FINAL TIPS TO KEEP SKIN TAUT AND YOUTHFUL

Skin does change with time. However, there are some things we can do to help skin retain its youthful resiliency, suppleness, and glow. Who doesn't want younger-looking skin? Here are a few tips to help you keep what you already have—and even restore a bit of what has been taken away:

- Avoid rapid weight gains and losses. Over time, the skin loses the ability to stretch and spring back. Repeated crash dieting is one of the worst offenders in the cellulite story. Rippling of the skin is a heavy price to pay for temporary weight loss.
- Keep your skin "active" with the methods described in this chapter. Regular brushing and self-massage will help keep skin fresh and youthful.
- Exercise regularly. This goes without saying, but keep in mind that skin reaps the benefits, too. Studies show that the thickness and elasticity of skin are actually enhanced with regular exercise.
- Consider more vitamin C in your diet. This important vitamin helps develop collagen.
- Try to maintain a good fat-to-lean ratio. By maintaining muscle mass and minimizing body fat, you are less likely to be affected by gravity's pull.
- Treat your skin gently. Unnecessary pulling and tugging will eventually take their toll. This, of course, holds true for applying makeup, creams, and masques to the face, but handle your body with a light touch as well. When using a body lotion, always apply with firm but gentle, even, upward strokes and apply on damp skin.

8

Stress Management
and Visualization

THE MIND-BODY CONNECTION

The mind exerts limitless power over the body. Were we able to harness and direct a fraction of our mental energy, we could all accomplish wondrous things. If we could channel this energy into positive events, we could actually control many aspects of our health, vitality, level of fitness—and the way we look. This is not idle speculation nor is it wishful thinking.

Scientists have only recently begun to probe the powerful relationship that exists between what we think and the realities we create. Our health, we know now, depends to a very large extent upon positive attitudes toward our bodies and our lives in general. Much evidence has collected in recent years to support theories of self-healing with dramatic recoveries from life-threatening illnesses and debilitating handicaps.

Our goal here is to improve physiology. A significant part of this can be accomplished with the mind. In a very real sense, this is where it all begins. Every plan of action that is set into motion begins with a simple decision. This is the first step toward overcoming a problem or a bad habit and the first step toward making improvements in any area. It is that initial "spark" ignited by mental energy that gives shape and sub-

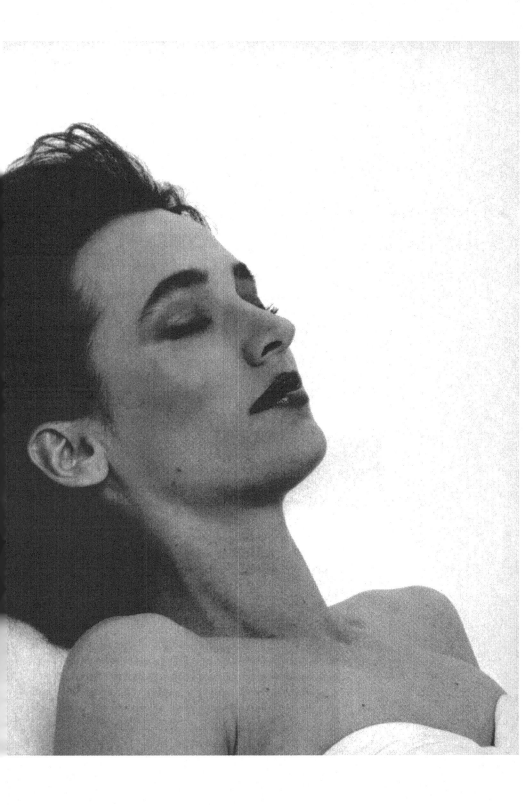

stance to practically everything we accomplish. This is no less true in the case of improving the body.

When we learn to manage the stress and strains of everyday life, we minimize the harmful effects that anxiety exerts. Wear and tear on the system is significantly reduced, and the vicious cycle of "stress creating more stress" is brought to a halt. By practicing time-proven relaxation techniques, we not only alleviate stress but we gain a sense of serenity that automatically carries into daily life. Finally, visualization, a technique that has been used by countless thousands of people—from world-class artists to Olympic athletes—enables us to bring physical reality into harmony with mental imagery.

The techniques in this chapter will give you that extra "edge" in your struggle against cellulite and in attaining the figure you have always desired. There is nothing mysterious about all this. By programming the mind, the behaviors that are necessary—eating right, exercising regularly, skin workout—will become habitually and pleasantly integrated parts of your daily routine. By implanting ideas and images, you will soon find that action automatically follows. Results will come more easily and without the frustrating "start and stop" that we often experience when we take on a new program.

STRESS: THE INVISIBLE ENEMY

Stress is an unavoidable component of life. No one is exempt from its influence or immune to its potentially devastating effects. Even in the most privileged of lives, stress can intrude and create chaos. It is an inevitable and inescapable feature of human experience. But while it can set our nerves on edge and our physiology in a frenzy, it can also have its positive side, impelling us to action by presenting us with challenges. How much it upsets our equilibrium depends to a large degree upon how we perceive stress and how we handle it. The various ways in which we cope with stress and anxiety have a tremendous influence on our mental and physical health—and on our figures.

Our looks are a reflection of our mental health. No matter how scrupulously we care for our bodies and how impeccably we groom ourselves, if we feel defeated, devitalized, and depressed, we show it. Physical beauty equates with mental well-being: confidence, fulfillment, and a joy in living will make the plainest of us positively radiant.

Stress is one of the most persistent antagonists to our health and our looks. This is true not only while we are in its immediate grip but in the long run as well. Controlling or managing stress is critically important in improving physiology, in restoring harmony in the body. Our goal in stress control is actually twofold: to make an ally of stress by learning to use it to our advantage, and to minimize its potentially damaging effects when it threatens to overwhelm us. By coping effectively with stress, we cultivate one of the most valuable assets we can possibly possess.

A life without stress would be quite boring. All of us require a certain amount of it to keep us on our toes. Dr. Hans Selye, the renowned pioneer of stress studies, called it "the spice of life" and identified "optimum stress levels," which vary from person to person and determine whether a strain will have positive or negative effects. It is important to assess how much stress you can handle successfully, whether the stress you experience is of a positive or a negative kind, and to prevent a stress overload from becoming a serious problem.

When our reserves of vital energy are depleted by the "bad" kinds of stress, we become vulnerable to a multitude of devastating effects. We are at serious risk as targets of hypertension, chronic fatigue, steady erosion of all bodily systems, and early aging. Obviously, we should take every measure to protect ourselves from these debilitating and possibly deadly consequences. No matter how hectic and demanding our lives or our work may be, we do not have to set ourselves up as the victims of stress. Controlling stress not only makes us feel calmer, it makes us feel more in charge of every aspect of life.

Contrary to what most of us think, it is not just the major crises and big pressures that overload us with stress. It is the irritations of everyday life, repeated over and over, that gnaw away at our psyches and erode our bodies. When anger, worry, frustration, and hatred become our abiding companions, we are doomed to suffer relentless stress. It is these "stressors," as Dr. Selye called them, that cause health to deteriorate and depression to set in. Learning to cope with these lurking saboteurs— traffic jams, broken appointments, canceled plans, deadlines, telephones that never stop ringing, long lines at checkout counters, and so on—is really the secret of better mental and physical health.

The body responds to stress by releasing certain chemicals—the stress hormones—into the bloodstream. Blood pressure rises along with blood sugar levels, blood vessels constrict in some areas and dilate in others, and most digestive activities slow or stop altogether. All of these changes in body chemistry lead to the familiar sensations of increased irritability, shortness of breath, quick temper, tension headache, sudden fatigue, and uneasy stomach.

When the stressful situation subsides and the state of alarm declines, our glands secrete the calming hormones that allow the body to return to normal. But when this cycle is repeated over and over, we are left in a state of exhaustion with serious consequences to our health. It's been estimated that over 75 percent of all disease is stress related. Our appearance also suffers: chronic strain leaves a trail of frown lines, pallor, and premature aging—and cellulite.

THE STRESS-CELLULITE CONNECTION

All the systems of the body are interrelated. A disturbance in one area will automatically set off a chain reaction throughout the body. The stress and tension pattern, a chief culprit in the cellulite story, is a perfect example of this. Delicate bodily rhythms are severely disrupted by stress, tension, and anxiety.

While most people can easily recognize that poor eating habits can be responsible for cellulite, they find it difficult to understand that tension is equally responsible. When you are tense and anxious, all of the major functions of the body are altered. Breathing becomes shallow. Circulation is impeded. Digestion becomes sluggish. Elimination is disturbed. Glandular functions are affected. All of these throw the body out of balance and set the ground for cellulite to form.

Chronic stress actually wears down the adrenals. While these glands are well known as producers of adrenaline, the "fight or flight" hormone, it is a lesser known fact that they regulate water balance in the body. This is a critical factor in the cellulite pattern. Unstable adrenal activity leads to a sodium-potassium imbalance because the delicate mechanism that regulates this process is thrown out of whack. As a result, the sodium-potassium pumps can no longer function properly. Now we have a cycle in progress: overworked adrenals lead to a mineral imbalance that puts the body under more stress. If you are eating too much salt to begin with, sodium retention will be even greater as will potassium depletion.

By wearing down the body, stress creates more stress. For many, sleeplessness becomes an all too familiar pattern, and a lack of refreshing, restorative sleep leads to fatigue. Insufficient oxygen intake in the body, caused by irregular breathing, disrupts cell metabolism and also creates fatigue. Blood vessels become constricted, cutting off circulation in the extremities. All of these malfunctions result in greater stress as the body becomes more vulnerable, less resilient.

When our physiology is thrown out of balance in this way, through the vicious cycle of stress-producing-stress, delicate body chemistry changes occur. This, of course, leads directly to disruptions in our internal environment, which, in turn, leads to lumpy cellulite.

SOME VALUABLE TIPS FOR MINIMIZING STRESS

Each of us has a unique "stress profile." Some are unusually susceptible to problems in relationships with families, friends, and colleagues—and the conflict, guilt, anger, and personality clashes that often ensue. Others are plagued with financial worries, career frustrations, and social pressures. Still others are tormented with a sense of failure or threatened by endless boredom. All of these problems are part of the stress syndrome.

To control stress, rather than allow it to control us, we must first sort out positive stressors from negative ones. The good kind of stress comes from situations that you view as demanding or challenging: This form of stimulation can arouse your curiosity and engage your sense of commitment. You will actually gain a greater control over your life by rising to the challenge. Negative stress generally increases your feelings of frustration, alienation, and helplessness.

It is the negative brand of stress that we must try to overcome or minimize by establishing certain habits. The following suggestions may serve as guidelines in managing or reducing the stress in your life.

- Experience is the best measure of what will work for you. Learn to draw upon your own resources in order to determine what you can change in a given situation. Sometimes, when a stressful set of circumstances cannot be altered, it is best to step back and reassess your position.
- Offset the negative effects of stress with more exercise. Stress is often a highly physical response that can be countered with vigorous, sustained activity. By releasing nervous energy in this way, you will accomplish several things at once. The body will return to normal more quickly through this kind of productive release as opposed to "fits of temper," which tend to be self-perpetuating and counterproductive. You will increase vitality that will enable you to deal more efficiently with the real causes of stress. An aerobic form of exercise such as swimming or bicycling will keep the cardiovascular system in prime shape. Slower stretching types of exercise, such as yoga and t'ai chi will induce a calmer, more "centered" feeling.
- Avoid adding extra stress to your system. Caffeine, alcohol, ciga-

rettes, and tranquilizers all have one thing in common: They are deceptive coping devices that will compound your stress by tampering with your nervous system. While these "drugs" may offer the shelter of temporary respite, in the long run you risk far more than you gain.

- Try to make time and space for yourself. In a hectic, demanding life, this may seem like an extravagant luxury, but it is essential to your well-being. Each day, set aside time for yourself, away from everyone else's demands. Use this time to read, think, relax, listen to music, or nap.

- Manage your time wisely. Some people benefit from making lists for each day or week. This should not mean that you are rigidly ruled by an inescapable structure, but by setting priorities and accomplishing tasks in a productive order, you can gain more unencumbered free time. A sense of accomplishment will do wonders to enrich those hours set aside for leisure.

- Try to do things one at a time. No one benefits from a senseless flurry of activity. When a task seems almost insurmountable, try to divide it into steps or stages. By focusing on a single phase of a task or a job before moving on to the next phase, accomplishments mount more quickly and with less apparent effort. You will gain a greater mastery over the task as you dispel that terrible feeling of being overwhelmed.

- Avoid eating under tense conditions. Because digestion becomes literally impossible when you are angry or highly emotional, eating will only make matters worse. You will not benefit from the nutrients in food under these circumstances, and you may actually experience indigestion and stomachaches. There is, for some, the added danger of bingeing when nervous and anxious. It is best to wait until you are calm—and you can eat slowly with a sense of relaxed pleasure.

- Always try to get enough sleep. This is essential in helping your body do its job of repairing, renewing, restoring, and replenishing. When you lie down, make a special effort to shut out worry, fear, and anxiety—these hostile bedfellows can be ousted with a little practice. Make certain that your bedroom is comfortably cool (fresh air is best), dark, and quiet.

- Be optimistic. When you are in a positive frame of mind, you are better equipped to judge even the most dramatic situations with a sense of distance. This will enable you to make decisions more wisely. If you have things to look forward to and goals to accomplish, you will be less distracted by problems.

RELAXATION TECHNIQUES TO HELP YOU DE-STRESS

Stress and relaxation are really two sides of the same issue. There are times when all of us feel the need to shut out stress at will and move into a state of deep and restorative serenity. This is not an optional luxury; it is an absolute necessity if we are to conquer the effects of stress. The benefits that we gain from relaxation techniques extend well beyond the short period of time required for their practice. While it is true that inducing a state of calmness has its immediate benefits, what we gain in the long run can affect our lives in very positive ways.

When practiced regularly, once or twice a day, these simple relaxation techniques enable you to summon reserves of vital energy. By devoting only minutes a day to systematic relaxation, you will find that irritability is sharply reduced, anger less easily provoked, frustration resistance is strengthened, and the general feeling of panic less easily brought about. You will discover quite happily that you are more resilient when a crisis strikes, more graceful in the throes of pressure, and better equipped in general when faced with life's little irritations. Overall, your sense of tranquillity will be enhanced steadily while feelings of anxiety fade away more easily.

Relaxation is a required prelude to visualization. It is important to keep in mind that you should not force relaxation; instead, allow it to come gently, easily. You may want to try all three of the following techniques a few times before you choose the one you'll practice every day. Or you may find that a combination works best for you. It is very important not to worry about how well you are doing. Try to assume a passive attitude. If your mind wanders, just bring it back and continue. Let relaxation happen naturally.

The Relaxation Response

Developed by Dr. Herbert Benson, a cardiologist at Harvard University School of Medicine, this simple mental exercise will put you in a relaxed but highly energized state in a matter of minutes.

How to Do It

Sit quietly in a chair where you will not be disturbed. Close your eyes. "Warm up" by concentrating on releasing tension from all your muscles, beginning with the feet and moving up to the face. Feel yourself becoming loose and limp. Breathe slowly and naturally. As you breathe in through your nose, try to be aware of the air as it enters your body. As you breathe out, say a word such as "one" (this can be any word that you select) silently to yourself. This is the technique: Breathe in . . . breathe out . . . "one." Continue this for about ten minutes. Then, open your eyes slowly and remain still for another minute or so before getting up.

This very efficient technique can be incorporated into any phase of your daily routine. Many have used it while commuting by bus or train, and it is a perfect exercise to do right at your desk. You will feel remarkably renewed when you emerge from the relaxation state, ready to tackle just about anything that comes your way.

Classic Relaxation Method

This method of achieving total relaxation of mind and body has been used for many years with impressive results. Like the Relaxation Response, it may be used any time you feel a need to let go of tension and achieve a profound sense of serenity.

How to Do It

Lie flat on your back on a firm surface such as a carpeted floor or an exercise mat. Close your eyes. Place your arms straight along your body with hands in a half-open position. Keep your legs slightly apart with toes pointed outward.

Begin by concentrating on your toes and trying to "feel" them without moving them. Command them to relax. Next, do the same for your feet to the exclusion of other body parts. Relish the feeling of limpness. Next, the ankles. In this manner, you work all the way up: legs, knees, thighs, abdomen, buttocks, back, chest, hands, arms, shoulders, neck, and finally the face—mouth, eyes, forehead. Every part, in succession, will feel limp and quite heavy. As you are enjoying this sensation of heaviness, try to clear your mind, reducing thoughts to an absolute minimum. Focus on something pleasant as you breathe slowly and deeply. After a few minutes, you will be totally and blissfully relaxed.

Autogenic Training

Developed in 1932 by Dr. Johannes Schultz, a German psychotherapist, this technique is surely one of the most pleasant and satisfying ways to influence the body with the power of suggestion. For more than fifty years, it has been practiced widely in Europe and Russia, yet it is little known in this country.

Autogenic Training teaches a form of "passive concentration" that allows mind and body to "self-regulate" toward a more harmonious state. This technique is particularly suitable to our purpose as it is directly oriented toward enhancing physiology.

A ten-minute session of Autogenic Training will leave you supremely calm and wonderfully refreshed. The more regularly you undertake these exercises, the more easily you will achieve the desired results.

In the beginning, you should devote only about one minute to the first exercise. After a few days, add the second formula. Continue in this manner until you include all six formulas in your sessions, adding them one at a time. Ideally, you should be able to produce the desired feeling before adding the next formula. Once you have mastered the technique, you will be able to bring about the relaxed, attentive autogenic state in a matter of minutes—any place, any time, under any circumstances. Autogenic Training is perfect preparation for the visualization exercises that follow as it increases receptivity to images and affirmations.

How to Do It

Seek out a quiet place where you will not be disturbed. Sit in a comfortable chair with good back support or lie on a bed or carpeted floor with your arms at your sides. If you sit, keep your feet apart on the floor, your back straight, and your arms relaxed in your lap or at your sides. Keep your eyes closed throughout the exercise. Relaxation is the key to effectiveness here—the less you force results the better.

Autogenic Training consists of six short sentences that are repeated silently. You must pay close attention as you say these sentences so that each one will have its maximum impact on the body. To prepare, take a few deep, slow breaths. Try to exhale twice as long as you inhale. For example, inhale on a count of three, exhale on a count of six. Do this four or five times. Now you are ready to begin.

FIRST EXERCISE: HEAVINESS You are learning to induce a feeling of heaviness in your arms and legs to produce relaxation. Begin with your right arm if you are right-handed (left arm if left-handed). Say to yourself:

My right arm is heavy [six times]. I am supremely calm [once]. My right arm is heavy [six times].

The feeling of heaviness eventually spreads to the other extremities, but at some point you can add "My arms and legs are heavy."

SECOND EXERCISE: WARMTH This exercise is similar to the first but concentrates on feelings of warmth in the extremities. It increases surface circulation while relaxing blood vessels and capillaries. Say:

My right arm is warm [six times]. I am supremely calm [once]. My right arm is warm [six times].

THIRD EXERCISE: A CALM HEART This exercise regulates heartbeat. Repeat:
My heartbeat is calm and regular [six times]. I am supremely calm [once]. My heartbeat is calm and regular [six times].

FOURTH EXERCISE: BREATHING This exercise promotes slow, deep breathing. Repeat:
My breathing is calm and regular [six times].

FIFTH EXERCISE: WARMTH IN THE ABDOMINAL AREA This exercise calms the central nervous system, improves muscle relaxation, and increases circulation in the midsection. Say:
My solar plexus is warm [six times].

SIXTH EXERCISE: A COOL FOREHEAD This final exercise has a general calming effect. Say:
My forehead is cool [six times].

As you are coming out of the training session, flex your arms, take a deep breath, open your eyes. Never "leap" out.

Pointers

It is important to repeat the formulas verbatim but *not* automatically. You must say them carefully, with intention and emotion, so that each sinks into your consciousness. You may combine the suggestions with imagination.

The heavy/warm formulas often produce a deeply pleasant and drowsy state, which indicates that they have been well mastered. However, you do not want to fall asleep. If you have a tendency to doze off during this kind of deep concentration, then you should sit rather than lie down.

If your mind wanders, don't be impatient. Just try to redirect your thoughts to the formula. Deep and total concentration is the key to effectiveness, so if you find that you cannot concentrate, it is better to stop and try again later.

As you repeat the formulas, speak to yourself in an appropriate tone as the various sensations are created. With regular practice, you will find that the sensations occur more spontaneously.

As you become more experienced, you may simplify and abbreviate the formulas. For example, as you advance in your training, the key words—heavy, warm, and calm—will produce the desired sensation in moments.

VISUALIZATION

Visualization is a natural skill. All of us engage in visualization quite regularly even though we may call it by other names—daydreaming, fantasizing. We are all highly visual beings. Even our language is replete with expressions such as "picture this," "see what I mean," and "imagine that." And we all tend to filter reality through the mind's eye.

The value of visualization, also called "mental imagery," is now well established and documented in numerous studies. Today, visualization is used in a wide variety of areas from health improvement, pain control, and healing of diseases, including cancer, to strategic planning, problem solving, and performance enhancement, to name a few. And it is fast becoming an integral part of sports training.

We can influence physiology quite effectively through mental imagery as the mind is connected to every cell in the body through the autonomic nervous system. It is this system that controls most of our involuntary functions, including blood pressure, heart rate, digestion, and the production of enzymes and hormones. Through guided imagery we can also influence the autonomic nervous system to improve the shape we are in. By practicing effective visualization techniques, we can guide the body's systems back into natural harmony. Digestion, circulation, lymph flow, and cell renewal, among others, can all be improved significantly with consistent mental imagery. Strong mental pictures will also help us take the necessary steps to accomplish our goal.

There is nothing magical or mysterious about mental imagery. Before anything is realized, it is first created and nurtured in the mind. Artists, actors, inventors, architects, and businessmen use visualization instinctively. We all do this to some degree when we flip through the pages of a fashion magazine and imagine how we would look in a specific outfit or hairstyle. We also visualize when we replay in our mind how a particular meeting or date went. We do the same with interior design as we imagine how a room will look after the furniture is rearranged.

Effective visualization requires motivation, relaxation, and concentration. Motivation supplies the impetus to sustain our efforts. Relaxation is required to shut out all distraction and allow us to slip into a highly composed and receptive state. Through concentration, we hold images in the mind that, in turn, communicates them to the body.

Approximately nine-tenths of the mind lies below the level of conscious thought. In visualization, we communicate directly with the subconscious mind through a highly symbolic "language" of images. In doing so, we circumvent the analytical and critical processes of conscious thinking. When we tap into the subconscious with mental imagery, the "pictures" are transmitted through the pathways of the autonomic nervous system. Thus, we can program the various systems of the body to upgrade themselves and function more efficiently.

Visualization and affirmation are powerful methods of altering the body. Obviously, pounds will not mysteriously melt away, nor will lumps and bumps vanish into thin air. However, the visualization process provides strong reinforcement to guide the behaviors that are required to attain a smooth, ripple-free figure. Eating right and exercising regularly become much easier and more automatic when the subconscious mind is engaged in directing behavior. The powerful focus gained through mental imagery makes us more resistant to temptation, less likely to stray from good habits, and more fortified in the commitment to our goals.

The power that is released through visualization is enormous, boundless. Everyone is familiar with the ability of yoga masters and martial arts practitioners to control subtle bodily energies to achieve remarkable feats. This principle of energy has long been recognized in the East and has many names. The Chinese call it *chi*. For the Japanese it is *ki*. *Prana* and *kundalini* are two of its Indian names. In our culture, we usually refer to it as "life force" or "vital energy." Physicists have only recently begun to study the power of this principle and how it affects the body and the world outside the body.

There are a few things to keep in mind when practicing visualization:

- Images cannot be forced. Allow them to occur naturally and spontaneously. Much like daydreaming, this should be a very pleasant and highly individual experience.
- Always visualize yourself in the present. See yourself in the shape you wish to be in. This is a method of self-direction, not self-deception. Therefore, when you imagine yourself as you wish to be, you are giving yourself suggestions, directions, and positive reinforcement.
- You need not apply the exercises literally. There is no need to "memorize" them as they are written here. Because visualization is

a very creative process, you may use your imagination to vary the exercises to suit your needs.

- When visualizing, it is important to do so in as vivid and specific a fashion as possible. Being relaxed and focused provides you with great power, so tissue repair, healing, and health promotion can take place continually, as a constant part of daily life.
- Keep in mind the main objective: to improve tissue physiology by dissolving the congestion or tissue sludge of cellulite. You want to reestablish better functioning of the tissue and better metabolic activity at cell level, better nourishment as well as better lymph drainage. You want to speed up or encourage the cell renewal process so that damaged tissue is replaced with new, healthy tissue. The overall goal here is to direct the body to work more efficiently.
- Always remember that visualization is not a substitute for your diet and exercise measures. Rather, it is meant to be used in conjunction with the rest of the program to supplement, enhance, and reinforce just as it is used in medicine along with more traditional methods.

Visualization Techniques

It doesn't really matter which technique you use for visualizing. Here are some that you may vary according to your own imagination and creativity. Try them all and see which works best for you.

STEP ONE: Use Autogenic Training or some other preferred method of relaxation to reach a comfortable, receptive state.

STEP TWO: Once you are completely relaxed, begin to visualize clearly and concretely those parts of your body you wish to improve. Hold this image in your mind's eye. You can see it either anatomically or in symbolic terms. For example, to represent the cellulite formations, you may wish to visualize clumps of cells stuck together in a rigid, cementlike structure, the "glue" or ground substance.

STEP THREE: See the "glue" begin to loosen up, to dissolve. See it becoming more fluid. Visualize the area becoming more "active": imagine movement, exchanges between cells and surrounding fluid. Picture the fluid or lymph charged with loosened materials, the metabolic wastes and residues, being drained away toward the abdomen where they will be flushed out through the eliminative channels.

STEP FOUR: See the area getting healthier, cleaner, clearer, more supple. If there is excess fat, see the fat cells becoming smaller and smaller. See the whole area becoming firmer, sleeker, slimmer, smoother. See all the lumps and dimples being smoothed away. See the bulges decrease more and more until they are no longer there. Feel your skin pulling in tightly over the smooth contours.

STEP FIVE: Now, see yourself in the exact shape you wish to be: slim, firm, smooth, supple. See yourself glowing with health, vitality, boundless energy. Know that all of this is happening right now as you concentrate. Feel the happiness and satisfaction of reaching your goal, getting your body in the shape you have always wanted.

Before ending your session, tell yourself that your tissues will keep active until your next session. Everything will keep flowing better and better. See yourself engaging in this mental imagery regularly, staying awake and alert as you do it. Then breathe deeply a few times. Open your eyes and resume your activities.

Additional Visualization Techniques

Using Light
Visualize a ball of very bright white or golden light in your solar plexus. See this light extending, reaching out to the areas you want to improve. See it becoming brighter and brighter, permeating every single cell as it cleanses, purifies, and heals.

Using Color
Visualize the cellulite areas in color. For example, see them in a dark shade of red to represent the congestive buildup. See the areas gradually becoming lighter and lighter to signify that the congestion is dissolving. As the area changes from dark to light, see it reach a lovely tint of pink, which indicates healthy, improved tissue.

Using Your Hands
Place your hands lightly on the areas you want to work on. Visualize a powerful beam of light like a laser coming out of your hands and penetrating your tissues. See the beam as it breaks up and dissolves the congestion. Slowly move your hands until the entire area has been covered. Then, using controlled sweeping motions toward the abdomen,

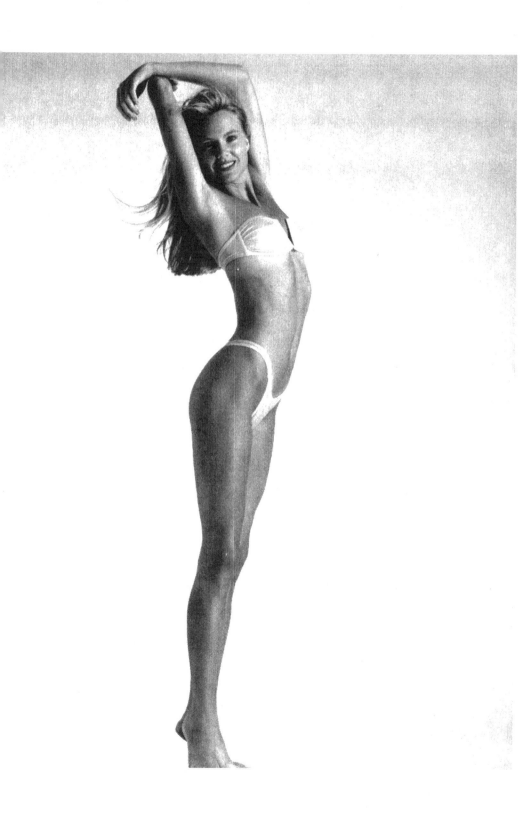

imagine your hands as magnets that collect and push along the loosened, dissolved materials. See these residues being drained away. Finally, see the area becoming firm and smooth.

Applying Visualization Principles

Visualization can be very useful in many instances. There is no reason to confine this powerful technique to your actual visualization sessions. You can use it to reinforce the other steps of your program. For example, visualize as you apply cream or body lotion. Imagine white energy as it penetrates your tissues, as it cleanses and renews. As you do this, see your skin as perfectly smooth and firm.

While exercising, see the area you are working on becoming firmer, more shapely. For example, see your stomach muscles glowing as they contract and fading as they relax. As you are walking, visualize your deep breaths as bringing purifying and nourishing oxygen to every cell, coursing through your tissues. When you exhale, see the oxidized, dissolved wastes being carried away. As you walk along, see your body, or a part of it, being firmed up, smoothed out. Feel the tautness. This last part becomes very easy because of the increased circulation that comes with walking motions.

Finally, feel the happiness, the pride, and the satisfaction that you will experience when you reach your goal.

AFFIRMATIONS

Visualization and affirmation go hand in hand. This technique of "inner speech" may be used along with visualization for added reinforcement. You may wish to use affirmations as part of your visualization session and/or as repeated reminders throughout the day, especially while performing routine chores or while exercising.

In affirmation, we use words rather than images to engage the mind in autosuggestion, which provides a set of instructions to direct inner processes. In this way, you program your own biocomputer to accomplish a particular goal. Just as some of us are more visual than others, some are especially inclined to respond to words. The combination of visualization and affirmation is most effective when tailored to individual needs and preferences.

Affirmations may be repeated silently over and over or written carefully in longhand a specified number of times—for example, ten to fifteen. The obvious reason for such repetition is to allow the message to "sink in." Affirmations should always be very simple, very clear statements that sweep away negativity and substitute positive mental directives. They are always brief and positive. Some examples may be: "My cellulite is dissolving," "My body is becoming smoother and firmer," "I am eating right and exercising regularly," "My muscles are firm and taut."

As you enter your affirmations in a notebook or on cards, or when you just repeat the words silently to yourself, do not do so mechanically. Instead, "feel" the meaning of the sentences, impregnating your mind with every word. Always construct affirmations in the present tense, as though you have already accomplished your goal.

You should reiterate these statements when you rise in the morning and again before you go to sleep. You may even wish to review or repeat them during the day as you're walking or swimming or stretching or doing housework. Remember, however, do not read or repeat your affirmations merely as a litany or a routine. Effective affirmation depends upon "feeling" the meaning of each statement. In this way, affirmations will become part of a powerful, influential mental dialogue with yourself.

Part Three SOME EXTRA HELP

It is important to keep in mind that the topics discussed in this section—the Fruit and Vegetable Cure, Reflexology, and Liposuction—are adjuncts or options that can be used in addition to—not instead of—the basic program.

9

The Fruit and Vegetable Cure

ere is a classic European method of rejuvenation and natural healing. Fruits and vegetables, as stated earlier, are invaluable in cleansing, detoxifying, and revitalizing the entire system. This *cure* is one of the very best ways to reestablish balance in the body while replenishing vitality, renewing clear mental focus, and brightening the spirits.

Most of us require the bodily equivalent of "spring cleaning" from time to time. The reason for this is simply that we tend to overload our systems with too many rich and processed foods; too many indigestible combinations; too much salt, sugar, fat, and protein. While it is not necessary to undertake the cure for your anti-cellulite program to succeed, I certainly recommend it for anyone who feels a need to restore overall health and vitality.

While it is true that the body is wonderfully equipped to handle the cleansing process on its own, we undermine its capabilities by the way we live. We add daily to the burden of toxic wastes, but we do little to assist in their removal. And through no fault of our own, we take in a great number of pollutants from the air we breathe and the water we drink. The result is more wastes than the body can reasonably handle.

This waste overload, along with poor circulation of blood and lymph, is largely responsible for physical and mental fatigue. Further, these wastes interfere with proper digestion and assimilation of nutrients. Water retention, puffiness, bloating, skin blemishes, and stiff muscles and joints can result. We suffer general subhealth conditions although we may not really be sick. Also, we encourage premature aging and the accumulation of cellulite.

It is virtually impossible to list all the wonderful benefits to be derived from this internal cleansing. Soaring energy and abundant vitality certainly head such a list. These are the natural rewards of efficient digestion, maximum absorption of nutrients, and the speedy elimination of wastes. Clearer, younger-looking skin, healthier hair and nails, and improved muscle tone are among the more visible benefits. Blood circulation revs up along with freer flowing lymph. And cellulite reversal gets a gigantic boost.

With this simple and natural process, we encourage the body to do what it would on its own if given the chance. The Fruit and Vegetable Cure literally gives it that chance. As we clear the accumulated wastes and dislodge toxic residues from organs and tissues, we clean up our internal environment and enable cells to function at peak efficiency.

Not only will the cure make you feel lighter and thinner (as you will probably shed a few pounds in the process, although this is not its main objective), but you will also gain an important psychological benefit. You will become more aware of the foods you eat and, as a result, become highly discriminating and ever more careful. You will be far more reluctant to put in the bad things—and far more eager to eat the foods that keep you in vibrant health and cellulite-free. For this reason, it is the perfect way to launch your new program of eating right, especially if you feel a need for an extra measure of discipline to change current habits.

Flexibility is one of the built-in features of this cure, and you may want to adapt the basic ten-day program to suit your specific needs. Maximum results, of course, will be derived from the program as recommended, but there are options for shorter "mini-cures." After experiencing this program, many people undertake it once or twice a year as a matter of routine. Others take advantage of quiet weekends for a three-day break from normal habits. Some prefer to extend the benefits by eating only fresh fruits and raw vegetables, and drinking their delicious juices, for one day each week or each month. No matter what option you choose, benefits will accrue.

There is a possibility of cleansing reactions as your body purifies itself. A rapid release of toxins may bring about dizziness, fatigue, headaches, and even muscle and joint stiffness. Not everyone experiences these symptoms, and there is no need to worry if you do as this is the body's natural response to inner cleansing. Should you feel headachy or unsettled, the best thing to do is rest calmly for a while in a quiet, dark room or practice the breathing techniques from Chapter 6 to accelerate the removal of wastes. Also, you should increase your water intake to help flush out toxins. Keep in mind that your body is using great energy to cleanse itself during this time, and you will not want to strain it further by exercising too vigorously. Easy does it on all counts while cleansing. Soon you will have energy to spare.

THE TEN-DAY CURE: HOW TO DO IT

If you are already eating well-balanced meals, you will be able to undertake the Fruit and Vegetable Cure without any special preparation. It is a more demanding routine, however, and you might want to consult a physician before beginning. If your current diet is heavy in animal products (meat and dairy) and processed foods, you will want to "ease into" the cure to minimize any unpleasant cleansing reactions. For at least two weeks before you begin, follow the principles outlined in Chapter 5 very carefully.

Here is the program designed for maximum results. During the ten days, you will want to observe the following:

- Eliminate *all* stimulants, such as coffee, tea (except for herbal teas), and alcohol. Except for prescribed medications, avoid any unnecessary pills, such as aspirin or tranquilizers.
- Upon rising, drink a glass of warm water with freshly squeezed lemon juice (half a lemon) or a cup of herbal tea with a squeeze of lemon. Do the same at bedtime. (If a sweetener is needed, use only the smallest amount of honey.)
- Drink plenty of pure water—at least *eight* glasses a day.
- Drink only freshly extracted fruit and vegetable juices—no juices from bottles, cartons, or cans.
- Be certain to eat slowly and chew your food extremely well. Sip liquids slowly.

Putting It into Practice

This program allows for five days of eating only *fruits and vegetables* (Days 1, 3, 5, 7, 9), one day of *fruits only* (Day 2), and four *supplemental days* (Days 4, 6, 8, 10).

Days 1, 3, 5, 7, 9: Fruits and Vegetables

Breakfast

This should be fruit, as much as you like: fresh fruit, fruit salad, fruit shake, or blenderized (puréed) fruit. It can also include a large glass of freshly extracted fruit juice. For the fruit salad, you may wish to add a dressing made from fresh fruit juice or fresh fruit puréed in a blender (fresh orange or apple juice combined with strawberries, raspberries, or pineapple). If you wish, you may choose to highlight a particular fruit—good choices would be grapes, pineapple, watermelon, mango, kiwi, or papaya because of their specific cleansing properties. All should be ripe. You should limit bananas because they are really a starch and will interfere with the cleansing properties of other fruits.

Fifteen minutes before lunch, drink a glass of freshly extracted fruit or vegetable juice.

Lunch

This meal may be a large vegetable salad in which you combine as many fresh vegetables as you like with a generous topping of sprouts. Half an avocado is a nice addition. A few seeds (sunflower, pumpkin, sesame) and nuts (almonds, pine nuts) can also be added. Dressing should be lemon juice and cold-pressed olive oil (safflower or sunflower oil may be substituted). Lunch may also include a raw soup selected from Chapter 5.

Fifteen minutes before dinner, a cup of blenderized fruit is ideal as is a raw soup. Or if you prefer, a large glass of fresh fruit or vegetable juice.

Dinner

You may wish to have another large vegetable salad for dinner, but vary the ingredients from the one you had for lunch as much as possible. Some other choices for a meal of vegetables would be a selection of lightly steamed vegetables (with a generous squeeze of fresh lemon) preceded by a fresh salad or an assortment of crudités. Another excellent choice for dinner would be a large fruit salad.

Note: Lunch and dinner are interchangeable in this program. Whatever works better for you.

If hungry, between these meals, you may munch on fresh fruits and/or raw vegetables—or drink their replenishing juices. However, please allow some time to elapse between servings as eating continually puts unnecessary strain on the digestive system. An hour or two is ideal.

Day 2: Fruits Only

Instead of eating conventional meals on this day, you should have fruit every two hours. All the alternatives above that pertain to fruit apply here: fresh, as a salad, a shake, blenderized, or juice.

Days 4, 6, 8, 10: Supplemental Days

Breakfast

This meal should be essentially the same as on Days 1, 3, 5, 7, and 9. Remember, these four days are still part of the cure, and eating a breakfast comprised of fresh fruits (in the form of your choice) will assure continuity in the cleansing function.

Lunch and Dinner

The emphasis here is on vegetables, but you need not have them all raw. Instead, you may include steamed or stir-fried vegetables with a small portion of grains such as brown rice or whole-wheat couscous or legumes such as lentils. Another choice would be a slice or two of whole-grain bread. The reason for adding starches on these days is to provide energy and to stave off the chilly feeling that may result from meals made up exclusively of vegetables. However, if you choose a cooked meal such as this, be sure to precede it with something raw such as a fresh, crisp salad, a raw soup, or a large glass of freshly extracted juice. Although you will want to avoid all animal products for the duration of the cure, on these days you may include small amounts of plain low-fat yogurt.

As you no doubt realize by now, potassium predominates in this cure—and for very good reasons. This valuable mineral, in substantial quantities and spread throughout the day, will spark the cleansing process and provide the "power" to keep it going.

On All Ten Days

- Be sure to include skin brushing—morning and evening.
- Practice the deep-breathing techniques outlined in Chapter 6.
- Exercise daily but moderately—thirty to forty minutes of walking is ideal, but you may wish to slow down the pace somewhat.
- Twice a day, lie on a slantboard for fifteen minutes or do a prolonged shoulderstand (at least five minutes).

These four steps will increase lymph drainage and greatly intensify the benefits of the cure.

SALTS BATH

You may wish to include this special bath two or three times during the cure, every other day for example. It's very simple yet wonderfully relaxing and effective.

Fill your tub with very warm to comfortably hot water to which two pounds of Epsom Salts have been added. Remain immersed for fifteen minutes as you massage your entire body beginning with the feet and working up. Dry off quickly and go directly to bed; keep warm as you will continue to perspire (perhaps with an extra blanket). This bath helps promote better circulation along with speedy elimination of wastes through the newly opened pores of the skin.

10
Reflexology

T his practice is both old and new. Many early civilizations, including the Egyptians and the Chinese, understood the principle of "energy zones" that run through the body, and it was for them a common practice to massage the hands and feet to balance the flow of bodily energy. Sometimes referred to as "zone therapy," reflexology has gained much popularity in recent years and now is regarded as a well-established technique with a multitude of benefits. A skilled reflexologist can make you feel absolutely wonderful from head to toe while improving many physiological functions.

What joins the ancients with the moderns is the belief that there are reflex areas in the feet that correspond to all the major organs, glands, and body parts. By stimulating these precisely positioned reflex points on the soles of the feet, corresponding organs and systems can be encouraged to function more efficiently and in greater harmony with one another. Put another way, reflexology helps Nature to normalize and enhance bodily functions in a perfectly safe, noninvasive manner.

Reflexologists specify that there are ten energy zones that run the length of the body from head to toe, five for each side, ending in each foot and running down the arms into the tips of the fingers. By massaging these reflex areas in the feet and applying pressure selectively through a series of "kneading" or "finger walking" movements, the reflexologist can determine which areas of the body require special attention.

The "map" of the feet illustrated below has been simplified to highlight the organs and functions that play a role in the elimination of cellulite.

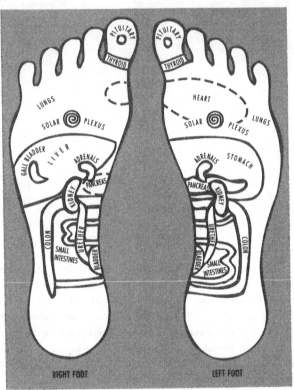

For our purpose of hastening cellulite reversal, reflexology will:

- "Tune up" the entire body so that it runs more smoothly
- Alleviate the effects of tension by inducing a state of deep relaxation
- Encourage more efficient functioning in circulation, lymph flow, digestion, and elimination, among other systems
- Help cleanse the body of toxins and impurities
- Decrease or minimize water retention
- Enhance glandular function
- Promote deep and restorative sleep

As with all massage techniques, reflexology is most effective when performed by a skilled professional. The high level of expertise that this person brings to the experience will no doubt give you the very best results. However, if you wish to experiment with reflexology in the comfort and privacy of your home, here are a few suggestions for a do-it-yourself version.

Sit in a comfortable position. Bring one foot over the opposite thigh. With the thumb of one hand, press the reflex points from heel to toe. After you have "thumb walked" the entire sole, give extra attention to the central area, which has a high concentration of reflex points related to cellulite. Then do the top of the foot using a series of "finger walking" movements from toes to instep. End your massage by working the lymph drainage points that extend from inner to outer ankle bone. Repeat movements for other foot.

Here are two final tips that will enhance the benefits of any reflexology session, whether professional or at home.

- Breathe normally throughout; inhale deeply and exhale forcefully from time to time.
- Following your treatment, drink a large glass of pure water to help flush away released toxins.

Should you decide that reflexology is an appealing and purposeful option in your cellulite reversal program, you may wish to consult some of the many fine books on this subject. These may serve to guide your decision for professional care while increasing the effectiveness of your at-home treatment.

11

Liposuction: What It Can and Cannot Do

Cosmetic surgery does have its place. For many women, liposuction has provided great incentive to achieve their ideal weight and has taken them a long way toward solving persistent figure problems. While it is certainly not a substitute for good nutrition and regular exercise, liposuction can give some women a more realistic starting point for launching a healthier way of life. And in some cases it may serve as a finishing touch for certain imperfections or distortions that would otherwise require superhuman discipline to correct.

Millions have benefited from liposuction. It is important to keep in mind, however, that many others have regretted the decision to "fix" their figures surgically. And still others have negated the effects of surgery by failing to confront the real causes of the original problem.

Despite its apparent simplicity, liposuction is neither easy nor miraculous. Above all, the technique requires a great deal of skill and experience on the part of the surgeon as well as a keen sense of aesthetics. It is wise to "shop around" for a physician not only by consulting a few or more candidates but by discussing the matter with former patients who are frank in describing their experiences. Bear in mind that liposuction can only be as successful as the surgeon who performs it.

The technique of liposuction is quite literally the sculpting of living tissue, and real artistry comes into play here. The results can be instantaneous and spectacular or quite disastrous—depending upon both the patient's expectations and the surgeon's abilities. Although scarring is minimal and recuperation is fairly quick, many other things can go wrong: Dents and hollows can result as well as other contour irregularities, and permanent distortions become a real risk if too much fat is removed.

For optimum success in liposuction, the patient must have good skin tone that is sufficiently elastic to adjust to the new contours once the excess fat is removed. Also, liposuction should not be regarded as the ultimate cure for obesity. The patient should, in fact, be within 5 to 20 pounds of ideal weight before the procedure is considered. It works best on specific areas of the body with localized excess fat. It cannot "shrink" the entire lower body.

The most common areas for liposuction are the outer thigh and lower abdomen. A skillful surgeon can work wonders in these problem areas by removing stubborn fatty tissue that may not respond to dietary or exercise measures—or at least not respond as quickly as one would like. Remember, however, that liposuction cannot smooth out unevenly textured skin. Cellulite, as we have described it and defined it, cannot be removed this way. At the time of this writing, it should be noted, new techniques are being developed to improve the skin's puckered appearance in various ways. Because these methods are still in the experimental stages, it is not possible to predict long-range results.

Age itself is not so much a factor in liposuction surgery as the individual's general health, weight, and skin tone. It is really a procedure designed to remove inches, not pounds. While the basic silhouette of the body can be greatly improved and clothing may be worn with new variety and in a much more flattering manner, the appearance of cellulite probably will not be significantly diminished. As I mentioned in the introduction, as of yet there are no miracle cures for cellulite. It remains a problem that is best and most effectively treated from the inside out. A surgical procedure such as liposuction, in some cases, may provide an excellent incentive for doing this.

If you understand liposuction's limitations and still wish to proceed with it, then remember to take great care in selecting a doctor who will give you the best results. Practice definitely makes perfect when it comes to this technique. Also, remember that your expectations must be realistic, and that the procedure works best when combined with the fundamental changes in lifestyle, which this book recommends.

Epilogue

W

ell, you are now equipped in every way to experience a life "beyond cellulite." You have all the "raw materials," so to speak, to transform not only your figure but your attitudes toward health, fitness, and vitality. The rest, as they say, is entirely up to you.

It is with my fondest wishes and my firmest promise that I offer this knowledge to you. By implementing it carefully and systematically, you will soon enjoy not only freedom from the imprisonment of heretofore stubborn lumps and bumps but a soaring sense of confidence that comes from knowing that you are now in complete control. Never again should you be tempted to succumb to passing fads and trends that leave you depleted of energy, discouraged, and, worst of all, back at the same starting point over and over.

Please remember to be patient. Now, in your effort to reestablish complete bodily harmony, you are on a new timetable: Nature's own. This is the wisest of schedules since it permits no false starts or desperate variations. Once you have begun to put this information into practice, your progress will be smooth and steady. Just think that very soon you'll be looking in the mirror with pride rather than a tinge of anguish. As you view your ever lovelier, healthier, stronger body, you'll marvel at the simplicity of the achievement.

I wish you *bonne chance* in your efforts—and I have the greatest confidence that your success will be accompanied by a fulfilling sense of joy.

Resources

NEWSLETTER

Mme. Ronsard is inaugurating a newsletter that will reinforce and expand on the book's concepts. It will also allow readers to have their questions addressed as well as keep them informed of the latest updates.

BEYOND CELLULITE—THE VIDEO

This new video highlights the practical steps of the program—nutrition, exercise, massage and visualization—and makes it the perfect companion to the book. If it is not available at regular outlets, it can be ordered by mail.

For more information about the newsletter, video and other resources write:

Nicole Ronsard
210 Fifth Avenue
Suite 1102
New York, N.Y. 10010

Index

adipose tissue, 3, 19
adrenals, 5, 164
aerobic exercises, 25, 85–86, 128–31
  bicycling, 129
  cross-country skiing, 130
  skating, 131
  swimming, 129–30
  walking, 128–29
  in water, 120–27
affirmations, 176–77
age, 5–6
  and teen-age years, 17–18
air baths, 154–57
alcohol, 10, 32
all-in-one exercise, 112–13
antacids, 14
antioxidants, natural, 71
arms, exercises for, 115–19
  bicep curl, 117
  finishing stretch, 119
  push away, 116
  triceps extension, 118
artificial sweeteners, 44
asparagus soup, fresh, 59

Autogenic Training, 26, 168–71
  pointers, 170–71

barley, 61
bath, salts, 186
Benson, Herbert, 167
beta-carotene, sources of, 71
bicep curl exercise, 117
bicycling, 129
bingeing, 5, 34
bioflavonoids, 72
bloating, 20, 45, 48, 182
body shaper exercises: See muscle
    firming exercises
body toxicity, 11
bread, whole-grain, 62
breakfast suggestions, 67–68
  high-energy shake, 68
breathing exercises, 26, 86, 144–45
  cleansing breath, 145
  replenishing breath, 145
broccoli soup, creamy, 59
brown rice: See rice, brown
buckwheat groats, 61

lunch suggestions, 68–69, 74
lymph nodes, 12
lymphatic circulation, xix, 11–12, 48, 86

manganese, sources of, 71
mango, for collagen renewal, 71–72
massage techniques: *See* skin brushing;
  skin, self-massaging
meal planning, 67–69
meats, 39
men, cellulite and, 6–7
menopause, 17
mental imagery: *See* visualization
microcirculation, 4, 10–11, 151
milk, 40
moderation, 24, 65, 81
muscle firming exercises, 26, 83–85, 88
  for arms, 115–19
  for buttocks, 104–108
  pointers, 89
  for stomach, 109–14
  for thighs, 93–103
muscles, gluteal, 5

nutrients: *See* individual names
nutrition: *See* diet
nuts, 63
  high in copper, 71
  high in manganese, 71
  high in vitamin E, 71
  high in zinc, 71

obesity, 19, 38, 43
oils, vegetable: *See* fats
oxidation radicals: *See* free radicals

papaya, for collagen renewal, 71
paprika, 72
pasta, 62
pelvic curl exercise, 110
pelvic tilt exercise, 105
pineapple, for collagen renewal, 71
plie exercise, 94–95
posture, 87
  poor, 15
potassium, 9–10, 48–51
  benefits of, 32
  menus sample of foods low in, 49–50

snacks low in, 50
sources of, 49, 50, 51
and tips for increasing intake of, 51
potatoes, 62
pregnancy, 16
premature aging, 5, 11, 71, 182
premenstrual bloating, 16
processed foods, 38–39, 181
protein, 40–41
pulsing, 95
push-away exercise, 116

quinoa, 61

raw foods, 37, 52–53
raw soups, 59, 195
reaches exercise, 90–91
reducing diets, 14, 23, 34, 159
reflexology, 187–89
  at-home treatment suggestions, 189
rejuvenation, 181
relaxation techniques, 167–71
  Autogenic Training, 168–71
  classic relaxation method, 168
  relaxation response, 167–68
rice, brown, 61

salad bars, 58
salad dressings, 57
  suggestions for making, 57
salads, 56–58
  suggestions for, 56–57
salt: *See* sodium
salts bath, 186
Schultz, Johannes, 168
sedentariness, 10, 14–15
seeds, 63
  high in copper, 71
  high in manganese, 71
  high in vitamin E, 71
  high in zinc, 71
selenium, sources of, 71
Selye, Hans, 163
shakes, high-energy, 68
sherbet, fruit, 76
shoes, high-heel, 16
shoulder stand, 146
skating, 131

About the Author

An internationally acclaimed expert in all aspects of figure control, French-born and -educated Nicole Ronsard can be credited for introducing and popularizing the concept of cellulite in America. Her book, *Cellulite: Those Lumps, Bumps and Bulges You Couldn't Lose Before*, published in 1973, provided women with an entirely new view of a figure problem that had previously lacked a name. The book was an immediate success and became a national best-seller.

Mme. Ronsard carried the cellulite message throughout the country on television, radio, in newspapers and lectures. Through her pioneering efforts, the term itself, common in Europe but unknown in the United States, became part of our vocabulary and forever changed our perception of the feminine figure. The word *cellulite* also entered American dictionaries and became permanently fixed in the language of health, beauty and fitness.

For the next several years, Nicole Ronsard continued her work in the treatment and study of cellulite. As owner of two Manhattan salons, from 1967 through 1981, she innovated various methods of cellulite control and body care that have since become popular from coast to coast.

Nicole Ronsard has spent the last decade further researching the underlying causes of cellulite and formulating new ways to combat it. This book, the result of her latest findings, will enable women everywhere to transcend cellulite for good.

Printed in the United States
by Baker & Taylor Publisher Services